Math for Healthcare Professionals: Dosage Calculations and Fundamentals of Medication Administration

Nancy DiDona, EdD, RNC-MN

Associate Professor of Nursing
Coordinator, Traditional Program of Nursing
Dominican College
Orangeburg, New York

JONES AND BARTLETT PUBLISHERS
Sudbury, Massachusetts
BOSTON   TORONTO   LONDON   SINGAPORE

World Headquarters
Jones and Bartlett Publishers
40 Tall Pine Drive
Sudbury, MA 01776
978-443-5000
info@jbpub.com
www.jbpub.com

Jones and Bartlett Publishers Canada
6339 Ormindale Way
Mississauga, Ontario L5V 1J2
Canada

Jones and Bartlett Publishers International
Barb House, Barb Mews
London W6 7PA
United Kingdom

Jones and Bartlett's books and products are available through most bookstores and online booksellers. To contact Jones and Bartlett Publishers directly, call 800-832-0034, fax 978-443-8000, or visit our website www.jbpub.com.

Substantial discounts on bulk quantities of Jones and Bartlett's publications are available to corporations, professional associations, and other qualified organizations. For details and specific discount information, contact the special sales department at Jones and Bartlett via the above contact information or send an email to special-sales@jbpub.com.

The authors, editor, and publisher have made every effort to provide accurate information. However, they are not responsible for errors, omissions, or for any outcomes related to the use of the contents of this book and take no responsibility for the use of the products and procedures described. Treatments and side effects described in this book may not be applicable to all people; likewise, some people may require a dose or experience a side effect that is not described herein. Drugs and medical devices are discussed that may have limited availability controlled by the Food and Drug Administration (FDA) for use only in a research study or clinical trial. Research, clinical practice, and government regulations often change the accepted standard in this field. When consideration is being given to use of any drug in the clinical setting, the health care provider or reader is responsible for determining FDA status of the drug, reading the package insert, and reviewing prescribing information for the most up-to-date recommendations on dose, precautions, and contraindications, and determining the appropriate usage for the product. This is especially important in the case of drugs that are new or seldom used.

Production Credits
Publisher: Kevin Sullivan
Acquisitions Editor: Emily Ekle
Acquisitions Editor: Amy Sibley
Associate Editor: Patricia Donnelly
Editorial Assistant: Rachel Shuster
Senior Production Editor: Carolyn F. Rogers
Marketing Manager: Rebecca Wasley
V.P., Manufacturing and Inventory Control: Therese Connell
Composition: Newgen North America
Photo Research Manager and Photographer: Kimberly Potvin
Senior Photo Researcher and Photographer: Christine McKeen
Assistant Photo Researcher: Bridget Kane
Cover Design: Scott Moden
Cover Image: © Helder Almeida/Dreamstime.com
Printing and Binding: Malloy, Inc.
Cover Printing: Malloy, Inc.

Library of Congress Cataloging-in-Publication Data
DiDona, Nancy A.
  Math for healthcare professionals : dosage calculations and fundamentals of medication administration / Nancy DiDona.
      p. ; cm.
  Includes bibliographical references and index.
  ISBN 978-0-7637-5843-1 (pbk.)
  1. Pharmaceutical arithmetic. 2. Medicine—Mathematics. I. Title.
  [DNLM: 1. Drug Dosage Calculations—Problems and Exercises. 2. Pharmaceutical Preparations—administration & dosage—Problems and Exercises. 3. Mathematics—Problems and Exercises. QV 18.2 D557m 2010]
  RS57.D53 2010
  615'.1401513—dc22
                                        2009002936

6048

Printed in the United States of America
13 12 11 10 09   10 9 8 7 6 5 4 3 2 1

I gratefully dedicate this text to my late sister-in-law, Geraldine. Throughout her illness, Geraldine encouraged me to write and to push myself to meet my target date. She never gave up her fight and was an example for me to emulate in overcoming obstacles and striving to make this book the best it could be. Thank you girly-girl. I miss you.

I thank my husband, sons, daughters-in-law, and grandchildren. Your encouragement and supportive words gave me strength. You are the air I breathe and the light of my days. I love you all. Thank you.

Contents

Preface

This math text will help users build their basic knowledge of mathematics and gain new abilities in solving complex calculations performed by today's nurse in practice and today's healthcare practitioner. The information is useful to a wide range of healthcare professionals, nurses, and allied health professionals who are responsible for unit dosing and client care outside the hospital setting. The ratio and proportion method is presented as the foundation for calculating medication dosages and intravenous solutions for clients across the life span and health continuums. This method is adapted to the dosage formula method and to the dimensional analysis method as a means of universalizing dosage calculations for all healthcare providers.

Many text features enhance the student's capacity to learn:

- Diagnostic test questions at the beginning of most chapters help users understand their strengths and weaknesses with regard to the chapter content.
- Sample questions are spread throughout most chapters at the end of each section of content.
- Practice test questions at the end of each chapter enhance users' understanding of their new knowledge and enable them to demonstrate proficiency.
- Illustrations throughout the text—such as medication labels, syringes and needles, IV fluid bags, IV pumps, and client chart documents—bring realism to the presentation.
- Two comprehensive examinations at the end of the text reflect the range of necessary math competency skills that the student needs to master.

Jones and Bartlett Publishers and I have worked hard to create a book that is user-friendly, informative, and an effective tool for the nurse or healthcare professional administering medications. Follow the book chapter by chapter, and complete the comprehensive exams provided at the end. Remember to look for helpful Medication Administration Tips, and information on classifications and uses for drugs mentioned in the text. We wish you the best of luck in your ongoing study and practice.

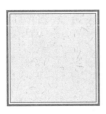

1 Basic Math Skills

Introduction

Each area of healthcare practice has requirements and expected competencies. This chapter is designed to assist you in

- Assessing basic math knowledge, values, and skills by working with various systems of measurement.
- Developing proficient aptitudes in basic math.
- Evaluating the application of basic math calculations.

Here are some general tips on technique and methodology:

- Try to solve the equations in this text without the use of a calculator and feel free to use scratch paper.
- Always reduce fractions to the lowest terms.

■ EXAMPLE:

$^4/_8 = ^1/_2$

- Solve all answers containing decimals to three places and round to two places.

■ EXAMPLE:

$18.737 = 18.74$

- As of January 2004, the Joint Commission determined there will no longer be trailing zeros after a decimal point.

■ EXAMPLE:

17.0 is to be written as 17.

- In addition, the Joint Commission requires a zero before a decimal point.

■ EXAMPLE:

.75 is to be written as 0.75.

Now take the following pretest. At the end of the test, score the correct responses using the answer guide provided at the end of the chapter. Add up the number of correct responses and multiply by 2. If your score is 90% or higher, you may choose to skip the review that follows in this chapter. If your score is less than 90%, please continue with the following math skills refresher.

Pretest

The following math problems are intended to assist you in assessing basic math skills and in refreshing your techniques in solving math equations.

Directions:

- Answer the following problems by filling in the missing information in the blanks.
- Use the space at the left of the page for scratch work.
- Remember to show all work and to proof all answers.
- The answers are at the end of this chapter.

1. 1 minim = _____ drop
2. 1 milliliter = _____ drops
3. 1 tablespoon = _____ fluidrams
4. 30 milliliters = _____ fluidounce
5. 6 ounces = _____ milliliters
6. 1 pint = _____ milliliters
7. 1 liter = _____ quart
8. grain $^1/_{120}$ = _____ milligrams
9. 0.4 milligrams = _____ grain
10. grain $^1/_{60}$ = _____ milligram
11. 1 grain = _____ milligrams
12. 15 grains = _____ gram
13. 8 drams = _____ grams
14. 454 grams = _____ pound
15. 2.2 pounds = _____ kilogram

Answer the following in decimal form. Remember to show all work and to proof all answers.

16. $^1/_4$ = _____
17. $^1/_2$ = _____
18. 0.5 + 3.25 = _____
19. 11.25 – 7.75 = _____
20. 6.5 × 2.4 = _____
21. 45.5 ÷ 5 = _____
22. $^1/_8$ = _____
23. $^1/_5$ = _____

Solve the following equations and reduce to the lowest form. Remember to show all work and to proof all answers.

24. $20\,^5/_{10}$ = _____
25. $^{12}/_{20}$ = _____
26. $^{15}/_{90}$ = _____
27. $^1/_5 + ^3/_5$ = _____
28. $^1/_6 + ^9/_6$ = _____
29. $^9/_6$ = _____
30. $^{25}/_7$ = _____
31. $^4/_5 + ^5/_9$ = _____
32. $^1/_3 + ^5/_6$ = _____
33. $^4/_9 - ^3/_9$ = _____
34. $^1/_4 × ^5/_6$ = _____
35. $^9/_{81}$ = _____

Convert the following numbers to Roman numerals. Remember to show all work and to proof all answers.

36. 170 = _____
37. 650 = _____
38. 35.5 = _____
39. 67 = _____
40. 23 = _____
41. 7.5 = _____
42. 1943 = _____

Solve the following equations. Reduce to the lowest form when necessary. Remember to show all work and to proof all answers.

43. 25% of 800 = _____
44. 60% of 720 = _____
45. 10 is what percentage (%) of 200? _____
46. 375 is what percentage (%) of 1500? _____
47. $^1/_2 + {}^1/_3$ = _____
48. $^7/_8 + {}^5/_{16}$ = _____
49. $^5/_9 - {}^2/_{18}$ = _____
50. $^7/_8 \times {}^1/_2$ = _____

Review of Systems of Measurement

The Metric System

For healthcare professionals today, the metric system is the primary method for determining correct dosages for medication administration. The metric system utilizes decimals, which translate into powers of tens. To increase a number, move the decimal to the right.

EXAMPLE:

To increase 10 (10.0) to 100, move the decimal one place to the right.

To decrease a number, move the decimal to the left.

EXAMPLE:

To decrease 100 to 10, move the decimal one place to the left (10.0).

Three common types of metric measurement are used in health care today:

1. Length, measured in meters
2. Volume, measured in liters
3. Weight, measured in grams

The basic units in the metric system have to be memorized and remembered for them to become familiar values.

M edication Administration Tip

The proper administration of medication depends on the nurse's ability to compute medication doses accurately and to measure medications correctly (Potter & Perry, 2005, p. 834).

Basic Units

In the metric system, the basic unit is incorporated into the title of every unit of measurement. All measurements of length contain the title *meter*, all measurements of volume contain the title *liter*, and all measurements of weight contain the title *gram*. The degree of length, volume, and weight is determined by the prefix attached to the unit title.

▪ **EXAMPLES:**

Kilo, denoting a large unit of measurement, may be placed before the title *gram*. When *kilo* (or its abbreviation *k*) precedes the basic unit, the basic unit is multiplied by 1000. A kilogram equals 1000 grams and is abbreviated kg.

Deci, centi, and *milli* denote smaller units of measurement. A meter is equal to 10 decimeters (dm), 100 centimeters (cm), and 1000 millimeters (mm).

Micro is another smaller unit of measurement. A milligram (mg) equals 1000 micrograms (mcg or µg). ▪

Abbreviations to Remember When Using the Metric System

Here are some volume and weight abbreviations to remember when using the metric system:

kg = kilogram	mg = milligram	mcg or µg = microgram
g = gram	L = liter	ml = milliliter
cc = cubic centimeter		

The Meter: Measurement of Length

The basic unit of measurement for length is the meter. It is equivalent to approximately 39.37 inches and is abbreviated as m or sometimes M. Nurses and healthcare professionals measure many physical findings for clients in meters, such as wounds, lacerations, incisions, drainage from dressings, moles, scars, and growths. Review the following units of measurement and corresponding abbreviations:

millimeter = mm = 0.001 m
centimeter = cm = 0.01 m
decimeter = dm = 0.1 m
kilometer = km = 1000 m

When converting from a smaller unit of length to a larger unit of length, move the decimal point to the left.

▪ **EXAMPLE:**

To reduce 1000 millimeters to decimeters, first count the number of spaces to move the decimal point. For this number, it is 2. Then move the decimal point to the left: 1000 millimeters = 10 decimeters. ▪

When converting from a larger unit of length to a smaller unit of length, move the decimal point to the right.

▪ **EXAMPLE:**

To change 50 decimeters to centimeters, first count the number of spaces to move the decimal point. For this number, it is 1. Then move the decimal point to the right: 50 decimeters = 500 centimeters. ▪

The Liter: Measurement of Volume

The basic unit of measurement for volume is the liter, abbreviated as l or L. A liter contains 10 deciliters, or 100 centiliters, or 1000 milliliters. The milliliter (ml) is equivalent to the cubic centimeter (cc), although ml is the preferred abbreviation.

Whether converting from a larger unit of volume to a smaller unit or from a smaller unit of volume to a larger unit, the system for moving the decimal point is the same as for length.

■ EXAMPLES:

1010 milliliters = 1.01 liters
5.5 liters = 5500 milliliters   ■

The Gram: Measurement of Weight

The basic unit of weight measurement is the gram, abbreviated as g, gm, or G. One gram is equal to

- 10 decigrams (dg).
- 100 centigrams (cg).
- or 1000 milligrams (mg).

A kilogram contains 1000 grams and is equal to 2.2 pounds. (A pound is equal to 454 grams.)

When converting from a larger unit of weight to a smaller unit, or from a smaller unit of weight to a larger unit, the system for moving the decimal point is the same as in other systems.

■ EXAMPLES:

8.8 pounds = 4 kilograms
1000 milligrams = 10 decigrams   ■

Metric System Practice Questions

Fill in the missing information. Remember to show all work and to proof all answers.

1. 1 gram = _1000_ mg
2. 1 kilogram = _1000_ grams
3. 1000 ml = _1_ L
4. 4000 milligrams = _4_ grams
5. 0.6 grams = _600_ milligrams
6. 275 ml = _0.275_ L
7. 60 kilograms = _60,000_ grams
8. 250 ml = _0.25_ L
9. 3.5 L = _3500_ ml
10. 500 milligrams = _0.5_ gram

The Apothecary System

The apothecary system of measurement is one of the oldest units of measurement for mediation administration and is still widely used for prescribing medication. When documenting in the apothecary system, the symbol stands before the quantity and the quantity is written in Roman numerals. For example, a typical order for aspirin (acetylsalicylic acid, ASA) is written "ASA grain x." If the quantity is large or is to be written out, then writing the Arabic numeral before the unit symbol is acceptable, such as 10 grains.

M edication Administration Tip

> Acetylsalicylic acid (Aspirin, ASA) is an anti-inflammatory, antiplatelet, anti-pyretic, nonopiod analgesic used in the treatment of mild pain or fever.

When a medication displays the drug dosage on the label as apothecary, the metric equivalent is usually included. Two types of apothecary measurement are commonly used in health care today: weight and volume. The healthcare provider must have a working knowledge of these measurements.

M edication Administration Tip

> The nurse is the most appropriate healthcare worker to administer medications. The administration of medications to clients requires knowledge and a set of skills that are unique to nurses (Potter & Perry, 2005, p. 840).

Basic Units

The apothecary system's basic units of measurement are

- grain, abbreviated as gr, or dram, abbreviated as dr or **3**, for weight.
- minim, abbreviated as m or min or *m̞*, or drop, abbreviated as gtt, or fluidram, abbreviated as fl dr, for volume.
- ounce, abbreviated as oz or **3**, or fluidounce, also for volume.

> **Abbreviations to Remember When Using the Metric System**
>
> Here are some common abbreviations to remember when using the apothecary system:
>
> gr = grain   m or min or *m̞* = minim
> dr or **3** = dram   oz or **3** = ounce

Concepts to Remember with the Apothecary System

- The symbol of the unit of measurement usually is written before the quantity.

▪ **EXAMPLE:**   gr xv   ▪

- Fractions are often used when the number or dosage is less than 1.
- Lowercase Roman numerals are typically used when the number or dosage is greater than 1.

The Grain: Unit of Weight

The basic unit of measurement for weight is the grain, which is the equivalent of 1 grain of wheat. Abbreviated as gr, it is the same as 60 milligrams. Medications such as phenobarbital and aspirin are occasionally ordered in grains and supplied in milligrams. The nurse dispensing these medications is required to mathematically convert the prescription to ensure that the correct dosage is administered.

M edication Administration Tip

> Mathematical conversion within one system requires knowledge of the units of measurement and basic math skills (Potter & Perry, 2005, p. 835).

M edication Administration Tip

> Phenobarbital (Luminal) is an anticonvulsant, sedative-hypnotic used in the treatment of seizures.

The Minim, Dram, and Ounce: Units of Volume

The basic units of measurement for volume are the minim (m or min or $\mathcal{m}$), dram (dr or $\mathfrak{Z}$), and ounce (oz or $\mathfrak{Z}$).

- A minim is the equivalent of a drop of fluid.
- A dram is the equivalent of 4 milliliters.
- An ounce is the same as 30 milliliters.

Clients who are unable to swallow pills or tablets frequently take liquid medications. The amounts are usually small, and careful measurement is necessary to ensure accurate dosing.

M edication Administration Tip

> Some forms of medications include elixirs, lozenges, suppositories, suspensions, lotions, ointments, syrups, tinctures, and transdermal patches (Potter & Perry, 2005, p. 824).

Apothecary System Practice Questions

Fill in the missing information. Remember to show all work and to proof all answers.

1 ounce = 30 cc / 30 mL

1. 60 minims = __1__ fluidrams
2. 1 fluidounce = __8__ fluidrams
3. 16 ounces = __1__ pints
4. 32 ounces = __1__ quarts
5. 5 pints = __80__ ounces
6. 2 quarts = __64__ ounces
7. 1 minim = __1__ drop
8. 1 dram = __60__ grains
9. 2 ounces = __16__ drams
10. 1 quart = __2__ pints

The Household System

The household system of measurement has been used by healthcare professionals and the public for many years. It was developed to coincide with the many objects of measurement found in typical households: cups, bowls, spoons, and eyedroppers (see Figure 1–1). Over-the-counter remedies often come with plastic ounce cups and droppers for easy use by the general public. The application of this system of measurement has increased in importance as client care centers more and more around the home.

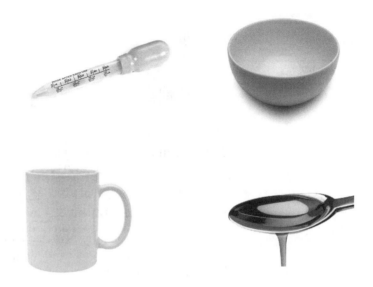

Basic Units

The basic units of measurement for the household system are the drop, teaspoon, tablespoon, measuring cup, pint, and quart. They are abbreviated as follows:

- drop = gtt
- teaspoon = tsp
- tablespoon = tbs
- cup = c
- pint = pt
- quart = qt

There is some disagreement among healthcare educators over how the apothecary and metric measurements convert to the household measurements. The approximate equivalents of household measures, metric measures, and apothecary measures are as follows:

Household	Metric	Apothecary
60 drops (gtts)	5 ml	1 teaspoon (tsp)
1 teaspoon (tsp)	5 ml	1 fluidram (fl dr)
3 teaspoons	15 ml	$^1/_2$ ounce (oz or ℨ)
1 tablespoon (tbs)	15 ml	4 fluidrams
2 tablespoons	30 ml	1 ounce
1 cup (c)	240 ml	8 ounces
1 pint (pt)	500 ml	16 ounces
1 quart (qt)	1000 ml	32 ounces

Household System Practice Questions

Fill in the missing information. Remember to show all work and to proof all answers.

1. 3 tsp = _____1_____ tbs
2. 2 tbs = _____1_____ ounces
3. 4 measuring cups = _____1_____ quarts
4. 1 pint = _____2_____ measuring cups
5. 4 quarts = _____1_____ gallons
6. 60 drops = _____1_____ teaspoons
7. 1 quart = _____2_____ pints
8. 3 tbs = _____9_____ tsp
9. 5 oz = _____10_____ tbs
10. 2 teaspoons = _____120_____ drops

Roman Numerals

Roman numerals are used in conjunction with the apothecary system of measurement. If the measurement includes a fraction, Arabic numerals are used for the fraction, with the exception of $\overline{ss}$, which stands for $^1/_2$. Remember, in the apothecary system of measurement, the unit symbol precedes the Roman numeral.

Table 1-1 shows Roman and Arabic numeral equivalents.

TABLE 1-1   Roman and Arabic Numeral Equivalents

Roman Numerals	Arabic Numerals	Roman Numerals	Arabic Numerals
I	1	XVII	17
II	2	XVIII	18
III	3	XIX	19
IV	4	XX	20
V	5	XXX	30
VI	6	XL	40
VII	7	L	50
VIII	8	LX	60
IX	9	LXX	70
X	10	LXXX	80
XI	11	XC	90
XII	12	C	100
XIII	13	D	500
XIV	14	M	1000
XV	15	$\overline{ss}$	$^1/_2$
XVI	16		

Roman and Arabic Numerals Practice Questions

Fill in the corresponding Arabic numeral. Remember to proof all answers.

1. XXIII = _____

2. MCMVII = _____

3. DCXV = _____

4. XIV = _____

5. CLXIX = _____

6. VII$\overline{ss}$ = _____

7. CDLXIII = _____

8. XXV = _____

9. IX = _____

10. XVI = _____

Percentages and Fractions

Percentages are very important in the field of health care. Many external medications, as well as intravenous medications and solutions, are written as percentages to express their strength. When working with percentages, remember that they reflect a portion of the whole, as compared to the whole, and that the whole is always based on 100. In other words, a percentage is a portion of 100. The percentage symbol (%) designates the measurement as a percentage. Percentages can be written as

- Whole numbers, such as 75%.
- Fractions, such as ¾%.
- Decimal numbers, such as 75.75%.
- Mixed numbers, such as 75¾%.

Changing Percentages into Fractions and Fractions into Percentages

To change a percentage into a fraction:

1. Drop the % symbol.
2. Divide the percentage number by 100.
3. Reduce the new fraction to its lowest terms.
4. If required, change the results to a mixed number.

■ **EXAMPLE:**

Convert 50% to a fraction.

1. Drop the % symbol: 50.
2. Divide the percentage number by 100: $50 \div 100 = {}^{1}/_{2}$.
3. Reduce the new fraction to its lowest terms: ${}^{1}/_{2}$.
4. If required, change the results to a mixed number.

■ **EXAMPLE:**

Convert 150% to a fraction.

1. Drop the % symbol: 150.
2. Divide the percentage number by 100: $150 \div 100 = {}^{3}/_{2}$.
3. Reduce the new fraction to its lowest terms: ${}^{3}/_{2}$.
4. If required, change the results to a mixed number: $1{}^{1}/_{2}$.

To change a fraction into a percentage:

1. Multiply the fraction by 100.
2. Reduce the new fraction to its lowest terms.
3. Change improper fractions to a mixed number.
4. Add the % symbol.

■ **EXAMPLE:**

Convert ¾ to a percentage.

1. Multiply the fraction by 100: ¾ × 100 = $^{300}/_4$.
2. Reduce the new fraction to its lowest terms: $^{300}/_4$ = 75.
3. Change improper fractions to a mixed number: 75.
4. Add the % symbol: 75%.

■ **EXAMPLE:**

Convert 7¾ to a percentage.

1. Multiply the fraction by 100: 7¾ × 100 = $^{31}/_4$ × 100 = $^{3100}/_4$.
2. Reduce the new fraction to its lowest terms: $^{3100}/_4$ = 775.
3. Change improper fractions to a mixed number: 775.
4. Add the % symbol: 775%.

Percentages and Fractions Practice Questions

Fill in the missing information. Remember to show all work and to proof all answers.

1. $^{1}/_2$ = _____ %
2. $^{1}/_4$ = _____ %
3. 12.5% = _____ (express as a fraction)
4. 56% = _____ (express as a fraction)
5. 33% = _____ (express as a fraction)
6. $^{4}/_{80}$ = _____ %
7. $^{25}/_{75}$ = _____ %
8. $^{5}/_{10}$ = _____ %
9. 16.6% = _____ (express as a fraction)
10. 40% = _____ (express as a fraction)

Conversion Within a System and Between Systems

Very often, when administering medications, the nurse or healthcare provider must successfully convert measurements within a system and between systems. To be accurate, the nurse or healthcare provider must memorize certain system equivalents. Table 1-2 lists equivalents between the metric, apothecary, and household systems. Remember that these are comparable values and not always exactly equal. Some calculations need to be rounded to accommodate medication dosages.

TABLE 1-2   System Equivalents

Metric	Apothecary	Household
—*	1 minim	1 drop (gtt)
1 milliliter (0.001 liter)†	15–16 minims	—
5 milliliters	1 fluidram (60 minims)	60 drops (1 teaspoon)
15 milliliters	4 fluidrams	1 tablespoon (3 teaspoons)
30 milliliters	1 fluidounce (8 fluidrams)	2 tablespoons (6 teaspoons)

(Continued)

TABLE 1-2 **Continued**

Metric	Apothecary	Household
240 milliliters	8 ounces	1 measuring cup
500 milliliters	16 ounces	1 pint
1000 milliliters (1 liter)	32 ounces	1 quart
1000 milligrams (1 gram)	grain XV	—
500 milligrams (0.5 gram)	grain VII$\overline{ss}$	—
60 milligrams	grain I	—
6 milligrams	grain $^1/_{10}$	—
1 milligram	grain $^1/_{60}$	—
0.2 milligram	grain $^1/_{300}$	—
0.4 milligram	grain $^1/_{150}$	—
30 grams	8 drams	1 ounce
454 grams	—	1 pound
1 kilogram	—	2.2 pounds

*No equivalent unit in the system.
†1 milliliter (ml) = 1 cubic centimeter (cc).

Working with Decimals and Fractions

Being able to work with decimals and fractions is an important ability in accurately completing mathematical calculations. Certain rules can help you safely administer client medications:

• When going from a smaller number to a larger number, move the decimal point to the *right*.

■ EXAMPLE:

$7.45 \rightarrow 74.5$

• When going from a larger number to a smaller number, move the decimal point to the *left*.

■ EXAMPLE:

$923 \rightarrow 9.23$

• When changing decimals to fractions, the number of whole digits to the *right* of the decimal point, which become the numerator (the top number), is equal to the number of *zeros* in the denominator (the bottom number).

■ EXAMPLE:

$0.421 \rightarrow {}^{421}/_{1000}$

• When changing fractions to decimals, divide the numerator by the denominator and place the decimal point where indicated.

■ EXAMPLE:

$^5/_8 \rightarrow 0.625$

Working with Decimals and Fractions Practice Questions

Fill in the missing information. Remember to show all work and to proof all answers.

1. 250 milligrams = _____ grams
2. 600 ml = _____ L

3. 0.5 g = _____ mg

4. 0.75 L = _____ ml

5. 1825 milligrams = _____ grams

6. 3000 milliliters = _____ liters

7. 4.5 g = _____ mg

8. 5.2 L = _____ ml

9. 0.1 g = _____ mg

10. 50 ml = _____ L

Change the following to fractions. Reduce the answers to the lowest terms as necessary. Remember to show all work and to proof all answers.

11. 0.25 = _____

12. 1.45 = _____

13. 0.5 = _____

14. 0.8 = _____

15. 5.6 = _____

Change the following to decimals. Remember to show all work and to proof all answers.

16. $^1/_2$ = _____

17. $^2/_3$ = _____

18. $^{10}/_{1000}$ = _____

19. $^4/_5$ = _____

20. $^1/_8$ = _____

POSTTEST

Remember to show all work and to proof all answers.

1. 1000 milligrams = _____ grams

2. 60 milligrams = _____ grain

3. 1 kg = _____ lb

4. 500 ml = _____ L

5. 1 tbs = _____ tsp

6. MCL = _____ (express in Arabic numerals)

7. 16 ounces = _____ measuring cups

8. 15 milligrams = _____ grain

9. 2.5 g = _____ mg

10. 16 drops = _____ minims

11. 10 kilograms = _____ grams

12. 4.6 L = _____ ml

13. 4 ounces = _____ drams

14. 1 quart = _____ ounces

15. 1 ounce = _____ tablespoons

16. $^4/_5$ = _____ %

17. $^5/_{10}$ = _____ %

18. 120 milligrams = _____ grains

19. 0.5 g = _____ mg
20. 2.2 lb = _____ kg
21. 36.5 = _____ (express as Roman numerals)
22. 1455 = _____ (express as Roman numerals)
23. 123 = _____ (express as Roman numerals)
24. DCL = _____ (express Arabic numerals)
25. XIX$\overline{ss}$ = _____ (express as Arabic numerals)

Answers

Answers to Pretest

1. 1 drop
2. 15–16 drops
3. 4 fluidrams
4. 1 fluidounce
5. 180 milliliters (1 ounce = 30 milliliters; 6 ounces × 30 milliliters)
6. 500 milliliters
7. 1 quart
8. 0.5 milligrams (60 milligrams = 1 grain)
9. grain $^1/_{150}$
10. 1 milligram
11. 60–65 milligrams
12. 1 gram (60 milligrams = 1 grain; 1000 milligrams = 1 gram; 60 milligrams × 15 grains ÷ 1000 milligrams)
13. 30 grams
14. 1 pound
15. 1 kilogram
16. 0.25 (1 ÷ 4)
17. 0.50
18. 3.75
19. 3.50
20. 15.60
21. 9.1
22. 0.125
23. 0.2
24. $20^1/_2$
25. $^3/_5$ ($^6/_{10}$ = $^3/_5$)
26. $^1/_6$
27. $^4/_5$
28. $1^2/_3$ ($^{10}/_6$ = $1^4/_6$ = $1^2/_3$)
29. $1^1/_2$ ($^9/_6$ = $1^3/_6$ = $1^1/_2$)
30. $3^4/_7$ ($^{25}/_7$ = $3^4/_7$)
31. $1^{11}/_{45}$ ($^{56}/_{45}$ = $1^{11}/_{45}$)
32. $1^1/_6$ ($^7/_6$ = $1^1/_6$)
33. $^1/_9$
34. $^5/_{24}$
35. $^1/_9$
36. CLXX
37. DCL
38. XXXV$\overline{ss}$
39. LXVII
40. XXIII
41. VII$\overline{ss}$
42. MCMXLIII
43. 200 (25% = 0.25 × 800 = 200)
44. 432 (60% = 0.60 × 720 = 432)
45. 5% (10 ÷ 200 = 0.05 = 5%)
46. 25% (375 ÷ 1500 = 0.25 = 25%)
47. $^5/_6$
48. $1^3/_{16}$
49. $^4/_9$
50. $^7/_{16}$

Answers to Metric System Practice Questions

1. 1000 mg
2. 1000 grams
3. 1 L
4. 4 grams (1000 milligrams = 1 gram, and 4 × 1000 = 4 grams)
5. 600 milligrams
6. 0.275 L (1000 ml = 1 L)
7. 60,000 grams
8. 0.25 L (1000 ml = 1 L)
9. 3500 ml
10. 0.5 gram (1000 milligrams = 1 gram)

Answers to Apothecary System Practice Questions

1. 1 fluidram
2. 8 fluidrams
3. 1 pint
4. 1 quart
5. 80 ounces (1 pint = 16 ounces)
6. 64 ounces (1 quart = 32 ounces)
7. 1 drop
8. 60 grains
9. 16 drams
10. 2 pints

Answers to Household Measurement Practice Questions

1. 1 tbs
2. 1 ounce
3. 1 quart
4. 2 measuring cups (1 ounce = 30 milliliters)
5. 1 gallon
6. 1 teaspoon
7. 2 pints
8. 9 tsp
9. 10 tbs
10. 120 drops

Answers to Roman and Arabic Numerals Practice Questions

1. 23
2. 1907
3. 615
4. 14
5. 169
6. 7.5 ($7^1/_2$)
7. 463
8. 25
9. 9
10. 16

Answers to Percentages and Fractions Practice Questions

1. 50% ($1/_2$ = 0.5 = 50%)
2. 25% ($1/_4$ = 0.25 = 25%)
3. $^1/_8$ (12.5 ÷ 100 = $^1/_8$)
4. $^{14}/_{25}$ (56 ÷ 100 = $^{14}/_{25}$)
5. $^1/_3$ ($^{33}/_{100}$ = $^1/_3$)
6. 5% ($^4/_{80}$ = 5%)
7. 33% ($^{25}/_{75}$ = $^1/_3$ = $^{33}/_{100}$ = 33%)
8. 50% ($^5/_{10}$ = $^1/_2$ = 50%)
9. $^1/_6$ ($^{16.6}/_{100}$ = $^1/_6$)
10. $^2/_5$ ($^{40}/_{100}$ = $^2/_5$)

Answers to Working with Decimals and Fractions Practice Questions

1. 0.25 gram
2. 0.6 L
3. 500 mg
4. 750 ml
5. 1.825 gram
6. 3 liters
7. 4500 mg
8. 5200 ml
9. 100 mg
10. 0.05 L
11. $^{25}/_{100}$ = $^1/_4$
12. $1^{45}/_{100}$ = $1^9/_{20}$
13. $^5/_{10}$ = $^1/_2$
14. $^8/_{10}$ = $^4/_5$
15. $5^{60}/_{100}$ = $5^3/_5$
16. 0.5 (1 ÷ 2)
17. 0.66
18. 0.01
19. 0.8
20. 0.125

Answers to Posttest

1. 1 gram
2. 1 grain
3. 2.2 lb
4. 0.5 L
5. 3 tsp
6. 1150
7. 2 measuring cups
8. $^1/_4$ grain
9. 2500 mg
10. 16 minims
11. 10,000 grams
12. 4600 ml
13. 32 drams
14. 32 ounces
15. 2 tablespoons
16. 80%
17. 50%
18. 2 grains
19. 500 mg
20. 1 kg
21. XXXVIss
22. MCDLV
23. CXXIII
24. 650
25. 19.5

Reference

Potter, A.P., & Perry, A.G. (2005). *Fundamentals of nursing.* St. Louis, MO: Mosby.

2 Organizing Mathematics for Medication Administration

Introduction

Utilizing an organized mathematical method for calculating medication dosages will assist healthcare professionals in administering drugs safely. The three methods discussed in this chapter are ratio and proportion, dosage formula, and dimensional analysis. The following pretest will assist in determining your proficiency in using the three methods.

Pretest

Solve the following equations. Be sure to label all answers, and remember to show all work and to proof all answers.

1. $\dfrac{1 \text{ kg}}{2.2 \text{ lb}} = \dfrac{x \text{ kg}}{540 \text{ lb}}$

    $x =$ _____

2. $\dfrac{1 \text{ g}}{1000 \text{ mg}} = \dfrac{x \text{ g}}{5600 \text{ mg}}$

    $x =$ _____

3. $\dfrac{1 \text{ grain}}{60 \text{ milligrams}} = \dfrac{x \text{ grains}}{15 \text{ milligrams}}$

    $x =$ _____

4. 15 ml : 1 tsp :: x ml : 7.5 tsp

    $x =$ _____

5. 1 milligram : grain $^1/_{60}$ :: x milligrams : grain $^1/_{10}$

    $x =$ _____

6. 100 mg : 1 ml :: x mg : 3.5 ml

    $x =$ _____

7. $x \text{ tablets} = \dfrac{1 \text{ tablet}}{0.25 \text{ milligram}} \times \dfrac{1.25 \text{ milligram}}{1}$

    $x =$ _____

8. $x \text{ ml} = \dfrac{5 \text{ ml}}{100 \text{ mg}} \times \dfrac{250 \text{ mg}}{1}$

    $x =$ _____

9. $x \text{ tablets} = \dfrac{1 \text{ tablet}}{50 \text{ milligrams}} \times \dfrac{25 \text{ milligrams}}{1}$

$x = $ _____

10. $x \text{ ml} = \dfrac{10 \text{ milliliters}}{100,000 \text{ units}} \times \dfrac{1,000,000 \text{ units}}{1}$

$x = $ _____

Approaches for Solving Mathematical Equations

Healthcare personnel approach mathematical equations in a logical and organized fashion in order to keep clients assigned to their care safe. This chapter discusses in detail the three most common methods for organizing medication calculations:

1. Ratio and proportion method
2. Dosage formula method
3. Dimensional analysis method

One constant with all three techniques is the need to know the equivalents of the units of measurement. Memorization of these mathematical facts is essential regardless of the process selected to solve mathematical equations.

M edication Administration Tip

Mathematical conversion between systems requires a comparison of the system of measurement ordered to the system of measurement available (Potter & Perry, 2005, p. 835).

M edication Administration Tip

Pharmacokinetics is the study of how medications enter the body, reach the point of action, and are metabolized and excreted by the body (Potter & Perry, 2005, p. 825).

Ratio and Proportion Method

The ratio and proportion method for calculating mathematical equations has been in use for many years. Some consider the method to be antiquated, and others regard it as a comfortable fit. It is mainly used to convert units of measurement within the same system and between systems of measurement. There are two acceptable approaches for setting up a ratio and proportion problem.

The first approach is to cross-multiply and solve for x. Given

$$\frac{A}{B} = \frac{C}{D}$$

cross-multiply and solve for x:

$$A \times D = B \times C$$

EXAMPLE:

$$\frac{1 \text{ tablet}}{500 \text{ mg}} = \frac{x \text{ tablets}}{1000 \text{ mg}}$$

cross-multiply: 1 tablet $\times$ 1000 mg $=$ x tablets $\times$ 500 mg
solve for x: 1000 $=$ 500x $=$ 2 tablets

The ratio and proportion equation is designed to solve for the unknown variable or x, which is placed in the numerator position. When setting up the equation, remember that like units of measurement must occur across from each other.

EXAMPLE:

mg (the numerator) is to ml (the denominator) as mg (the numerator) is to ml (the denominator).

The second approach is to multiply the means (the middle) and the extremes (the ends) and to solve for x. Given

$A : B :: C : D$

Multiply the means ($B \times C$) and the extremes ($A \times D$) and solve for x. This variation is used less than the first but is just as accurate.

EXAMPLE:

1 tablet : 500 mg :: x tablets : 1000 mg

Multiply: 500 x $=$ 1000
Solve for x: x $=$ 2 tablets

When you set up the equation to multiply the means and the extremes, the units of measurement appear in the same order on both sides of the equation: mg $\times$ ml on one side and mg $\times$ ml on the other.

M *edication Administration Tip*

Cross-multiply:	Means:
$\dfrac{mg}{ml} = \dfrac{mg}{ml}$	mg : ml :: mg : ml

No matter which version of ratio and proportion you choose to use, you must know the equivalents for the different systems of measurement (see Chapter 1).

M *edication Administration Tip*

To convert milligrams to grams, divide by 1000 or simply move the decimal point three spaces to the left (Potter & Perry, 2005, p. 835).

Practice Questions for Ratio and Proportion

Solve for x. Be sure to label the answer, show all work, and proof all answers.

1. 60 milligrams : grain I :: x milligrams : grain XVI$\overline{ss}$

    $x = $ _____

2. 1000 mg : 1 g :: x mg : 3 g

   x = _____

3. $\dfrac{1000 \text{ ml}}{1 \text{ L}} = \dfrac{x \text{ ml}}{0.5 \text{ L}}$

   x = _____

4. $\dfrac{15 \text{ ml}}{1 \text{ tbs}} = \dfrac{x \text{ ml}}{5 \text{ tbs}}$

   x = _____

5. $\dfrac{0.125 \text{ milligram}}{1 \text{ tablet}} = \dfrac{x \text{ milligrams}}{2 \text{ tablets}}$

   x = _____

Dosage Formula Method

The dosage formula method for calculating medication administration is an alternative to the less used ratio and proportion method. The three most commonly used formulas for medication and intravenous fluid administration are

- $\dfrac{D}{H} \times Q = X$

- $\dfrac{V}{T} \times DF = R$

- $\dfrac{TV}{TT} = HR$

Memorize

▪ **EXAMPLE:**

MD orders 1000 mg of a medication. On hand are 500 mg tablets.

Set up: $\dfrac{1000 \text{ mg}}{500 \text{ mg}} \times 1$ tablet

Solve: $\dfrac{1000}{500} = 2$ tablets

OR

▪ **EXAMPLE:**

MD orders 1 gram of a medication. On hand are 500 mg tablets.

Set up: $\dfrac{1 \text{ gram}}{500 \text{ mg}} \times 1$ tablet

Solve: $\dfrac{1 \text{ gram}}{500 \text{ mg}} = \dfrac{1000 \text{ mg}}{500 \text{ mg}} = 2$ tablets   *same*

*Note: The dose ordered must be converted to the dose on hand in order to solve the equation. In this example, the 1 gram was converted to 1000 mg because the tablets on hand were in mg.

■ **EXAMPLE:**   MD orders 1000 ml to run in 8 hours. Drop factor on the tubing is 10.

Set up: $\dfrac{1000 \text{ ml}}{8 \text{ hours}} \times \dfrac{10}{60}$

Solve: $\dfrac{10,000}{480} = 20.8 = 21 \text{ gtts/min}$

M **edication Administration Tip**

> Here is what the dosage formula method abbreviations mean:
>
> D = doctor's order
> H = on hand/available
> Q = quantity
> X = dose to be administered
> V = volume to be infused
> T = time needed to infuse intravenous fluid
> DF = drop factor (C = calibration may also be used.)
> R = rate of intravenous fluid administration in gtts/min
> TV = total volume
> TT = total time
> HR = rate of intravenous fluid administration in ml/hr

M **edication Administration Tip**

> To convert liters to milliliters, multiply by 1000 or simply move the decimal point three spaces to the right (Potter & Perry, 2005, p. 835).

To use the dosage formula method, select the formula required to make the necessary calculation, then substitute the letters for the values pertinent to the equation.

M **edication Administration Tip**

> A basic formula to use when calculating solid or liquid medication dosages is (Potter & Perry, 2005, p. 835):
>
> $$\dfrac{\text{Dose ordered}}{\text{Dose on hand}} \times \text{Amount on hand} = \text{Amount to administer}$$

Practice Questions for Dosage Formula

Solve for dosage. Be sure to label the answer, show all work, and proof all answers.

1. $\dfrac{500 \text{ mg}}{1 \text{ g}} \times \dfrac{5 \text{ ml}}{1} = $ _____

2. $\dfrac{120 \text{ milligrams}}{\text{grain I}} \times \dfrac{1 \text{ tablet}}{1} = $ _____

3. $\dfrac{100{,}000 \text{ units}}{1{,}000{,}000 \text{ units}} \times \dfrac{10 \text{ milliliters}}{1} = $ _____

M *edication Administration Tip*

> Medications, such as heparin, penicillin, and insulin, are supplied in units. There is no conversion to be completed as the unit is a unique measurement.

4. $\dfrac{1 \text{ gram}}{500 \text{ milligrams}} \times \dfrac{1 \text{ capsule}}{1} = $ _____

5. $\dfrac{32 \text{ units}}{100 \text{ units}} \times \dfrac{1 \text{ milliliter}}{1} = $ _____

Dimensional Analysis Method

The dimensional analysis method is a widely used alternative to the ratio and proportion and the dosage formula methods. There are no formulas to memorize with dimensional analysis, which is often referred to as logical and commonsensical. The steps to using the dimensional analysis method are as follows:

- *Step 1:* Determine the unit of measurement for the unknown in the equation. This value, usually written as *x*, may be expressed in terms of tablets, capsules, milligrams, milliliters, or any other unit of measurement. The labeled *x* is then written to the left of the equation and followed by an equals (=) sign.

- *Step 2:* Set up the rest of the equation to the right of the equals sign. This allows you to determine the dosage. In other words, the amount to give equals (=) what is on hand or available × what is desired/ordered.

▪ **EXAMPLES:**

$$x \text{ tablets} = \dfrac{\text{On-hand tablets}}{\text{Milligrams}} \times \dfrac{\text{Milligrams}}{1}$$

$$x \text{ milliliters} = \dfrac{\text{On-hand milliliters}}{\text{Grains}} \times \dfrac{\text{Grains}}{1}$$

- *Step 3:* Once you have the method written up, cancel out all units of measurement except the unknown *x*. Solve the equation. Your answer is with the only remaining unit of measurement on the left side of the equation. The numerator for the desired dose (the unknown) and for the on-hand amount must be the same.

▪ **EXAMPLE:**

$$x \text{ tablets} = \dfrac{1 \text{ tablet}}{500 \text{ mg}} \times 1000 \text{ mg}$$

Solve for *x*: $x \text{ tablets} = \dfrac{1000}{500} = 2 \text{ tablets}$

M *edication Administration Tip*

> Forms of oral medications include tablets (scored and unscored), capsules, gelatin-coated liquid, extended-release capsules, and enteric-coated tablets (Potter & Perry, 2005, p. 823).

Practice Questions for Dimensional Analysis

Solve for x. Remember to label the answer, show all work, and proof all answers.

1. $x \text{ tablets} = \dfrac{1 \text{ tablet}}{0.25 \text{ milligram}} \times \dfrac{0.125 \text{ milligram}}{1}$

   $x =$ _____

2. $x \text{ ml} = \dfrac{5 \text{ ml}}{2 \text{ g}} \times \dfrac{0.75 \text{ g}}{1}$

   $x =$ _____

3. $x \text{ milligrams} = \dfrac{1500 \text{ milligrams}}{3 \text{ tablets}} \times \dfrac{1 \text{ tablet}}{1}$

   $x =$ _____

4. $x \text{ vials} = \dfrac{1 \text{ ml vial}}{100 \text{ mg}} \times \dfrac{25 \text{ mg}}{1}$

   $x =$ _____

5. $x \text{ capsules} = \dfrac{1 \text{ capsule}}{500 \text{ milligrams}} \times \dfrac{1000 \text{ milligrams}}{1}$

   $x =$ _____

M *edication Administration Tip*

> To administer medications, the nurse must understand basic arithmetic to calculate doses, to mix solutions, and to perform a variety of other activities. This skill is important because medications are not always dispensed in the unit of measure in which they are ordered (Potter & Perry, 2005, p. 835).

POSTTEST

Solve the following problems using the three approaches for solving mathematical equations. Be sure to label all answers, show all work, and proof all answers.

1. *Ordered:* Codiene 30 mg PO STAT
   Supply: Codiene grain I tablets
   Give: _____

Ratio and proportion method:

Dosage formula:

Dimensional analysis:

2. *Ordered:* Potassium chloride (KCl) 20 mEq IVPB STAT
   Supply: KCl 40 mEq in 20 ml
   Give: _____
   Ratio and proportion method:

   Dosage formula:

   Dimensional analysis:

M edication Administration Tip

Potassium chloride (KCl) is supplied in milliequivalents, abbreviated as mEq. There is no conversion to be completed as the milliequivalent is a unique measurement.

3. *Ordered:* Prednisone 20 milligrams po TID
   Supply: Prednisone 5-milligram scored tablets
   Give: _____
   Ratio and proportion method:

   Dosage formula method:

   Dimensional analysis method:

4. *Ordered:* Tetracycline 100 mg intramuscularly BID
   Supply: Tetracycline 250 mg in 5 ml
   Give: _____
   Ratio and proportion method:

   Dosage formula method:

   Dimensional analysis method:

5. *Ordered:* Phenobarbital liquid 0.5 g po QID
   Supply: Phenobarbital 250 mg per ml in a 10-ml vial
   Give: _____
   Ratio and proportion method:

Dosage formula method:

Dimensional analysis method:

6. *Ordered:* Atropine 0.3 mg intramuscularly on call to operating room
   Supply: Atropine 0.4 mg in 0.5 ml
   Give: _____
   Ratio and proportion method:

   Dosage formula method:

   Dimensional analysis method:

7. *Ordered:* Lasix 40 mg IV push STAT and Q8H
   Supply: Lasix 20 mg per 5 ml in a 20-ml vial
   Give: _____
   Ratio and proportion method:

   Dosage formula method:

   Dimensional analysis method:

8. *Ordered:* Robaxin 0.4 g IV Q6H
   Supply: Robaxin 150 mg per ml
   Give: _____
   Ratio and proportion method:

   Dosage formula method:

   Dimensional analysis method:

9. *Ordered:* Stadol 1.5 mg IV Q4H PRN for pain
   Supply: Stadol 2 mg per ml in a 5-ml vial
   Give: _____
   Ratio and proportion method:

   Dosage formula method:

   Dimensional analysis method:

10. *Ordered:* Apresoline 15 milligrams po TID
    Supply: Apresoline 10-milligram tablets
    Give: _____
    Ratio and proportion method:

Dosage formula method:

Dimensional analysis method:

11. *Ordered:* Demerol 75 mg intramuscularly on call to operating room
    Supply: Demerol 100 mg in 2 ml
    Give: _____
    Ratio and proportion method:

    Dosage formula method:

    Dimensional analysis method:

12. *Ordered:* Benadryl 25 mg po Q4H PRN for itchiness
    Supply: Benadryl 12.5 mg in 5 ml
    Give: _____
    Ratio and proportion method:

    Dosage formula method:

    Dimensional analysis method:

13. *Ordered:* Regular insulin 15 units subcutaneously every morning
    Supply: Regular insulin 100 units per milliliter in a 10-milliliter vial
    Give: _____
    Ratio and proportion method:

    Dosage formula method:

    Dimensional analysis method:

14. *Ordered:* Heparin 10,000 units intrafat Q12H
    Supply: Heparin 15,000 units per 1 milliliter
    Give: _____
    Ratio and proportion method:

    Dosage formula method:

    Dimensional analysis method:

15. *Ordered:* Valium 2 mg intramuscularly Q6H PRN for agitation
    Supply: Valium 5 mg per ml
    Give: _____
    Ratio and proportion method:

    Dosage formula method:

    Dimensional analysis method:

Answers

Answers to Pretest

1. 245.45 kg
2. 5.6 g
3. grain ¼
4. 112.5 ml
5. 6 milligrams
6. 350 mg
7. 0.5 tablet
8. 12.5 ml
9. 0.5 tablet
10. 100 ml

Answers to Practice Questions for Ratio and Proportion

1. 990 milligrams
2. 3000 mg
3. 500 ml
4. 75 ml
5. 0.25 milligram

Answers to Practice Questions for Dosage Formula

1. 2.5 ml (500 mg ÷ 1 g = 0.5 g ÷ 1 g)
2. 2 tablets (60 milligrams = grain I; 120 milligrams ÷ 60 milligrams)
3. 1 milliliter
4. 2 capsules
5. 0.32 milliliter

Answers to Practice Questions for Dimensional Analysis

1. ½ tablet
2. 1.875 ml
3. 500 milligrams
4. 0.25 vial
5. 2 capsules

Answers to Posttest

1. *Answer:* ½ tablet

   Ratio and proportion method:

   $$\frac{1 \text{ tablet}}{60 \text{ milligrams}} = \frac{x \text{ tablets}}{30 \text{ milligrams}} = \text{½ tablet}$$

   Dosage formula method:

   $$\frac{30 \text{ milligrams}}{60 \text{ milligrams}} \times \frac{1 \text{ tablet}}{1} = \text{½ tablet}$$

   Dimensional analysis method:

   $$\frac{1 \text{ tablet}}{60 \text{ milligrams}} \times \frac{30 \text{ milligrams}}{1} = \text{½ tablet}$$

[handwritten annotation:] 1 gr = 60 mg

2. *Answer:* 10 ml

   Ratio and proportion method:

   $$\frac{20\ ml}{40\ mEq} = \frac{x\ ml}{20\ mEq} = 10\ ml$$

   Dosage formula method:

   $$\frac{20\ mEq}{40\ mEq} \times \frac{20\ ml}{1} = 10\ ml$$

   Dimensional analysis method:

   $$\frac{20\ ml}{40\ mEq} \times \frac{20\ mEq}{1} = 10\ ml$$

3. *Answer:* 4 tablets

   Ratio and proportion method:

   $$\frac{1\ tablet}{5\ milligrams} = \frac{x\ tablets}{20\ milligrams} = 4\ tablets$$

   Dosage formula method:

   $$\frac{20\ milligrams}{5\ milligrams} \times \frac{1\ tablet}{1} = 4\ tablets$$

   Dimensional analysis method:

   $$\frac{1\ tablet}{5\ milligrams} \times \frac{20\ milligrams}{1} = 4\ tablets$$

4. *Answer:* 2 ml

   Ratio and proportion method:

   $$\frac{5\ ml}{250\ mg} = \frac{x\ ml}{100\ mg} = 2\ ml$$

   Dosage formula method:

   $$\frac{100\ mg}{250\ mg} \times \frac{5\ ml}{1} = 2\ ml$$

   Dimensional analysis method:

   $$\frac{5\ ml}{250\ g} \times \frac{100\ mg}{1} = 2\ ml$$

5. *Answer:* 2 ml

   Ratio and proportion method:

   $$\frac{250\ mg}{10\ ml} = \frac{x\ ml}{500\ mg} = 2\ ml$$

   Dosage formula method:

   $$\frac{500\ mg}{250\ mg} \times \frac{1\ ml}{1} = 2\ ml$$

   Dimensional analysis method:

   $$\frac{1\ ml}{250\ mg} \times \frac{500\ mg}{1} = 2\ ml$$

6. *Answer:* 0.375 ml

   Ratio and proportion method:

   $$\frac{0.5 \text{ ml}}{0.4 \text{ mg}} = \frac{x \text{ ml}}{0.3 \text{ mg}} = 0.375 \text{ ml}$$

   Dosage formula method:

   $$\frac{0.3 \text{ mg}}{0.4 \text{ mg}} \times \frac{5 \text{ ml}}{1} = 0.375 \text{ ml}$$

   Dimensional analysis method:

   $$\frac{0.5 \text{ ml}}{0.4 \text{ mg}} \times \frac{0.3 \text{ mg}}{1} = 0.375 \text{ ml}$$

7. *Answer:* 10 ml

   Ratio and proportion method:

   $$\frac{5 \text{ ml}}{20 \text{ mg}} = \frac{x \text{ ml}}{40 \text{ mg}} = 10 \text{ ml}$$

   Dosage formula method:

   $$\frac{40 \text{ mg}}{20 \text{ mg}} \times \frac{5 \text{ ml}}{1} = 10 \text{ ml}$$

   Dimensional analysis method:

   $$\frac{5 \text{ ml}}{20 \text{ mg}} \times \frac{40 \text{ mg}}{1} = 10 \text{ ml}$$

8. *Answer:* 2.7 ml

   Ratio and proportion method:

   $$\frac{1 \text{ ml}}{150 \text{ mg}} = \frac{x \text{ ml}}{400 \text{ mg}} = 2.7 \text{ ml}$$

   Dosage formula method:

   $$\frac{400 \text{ mg}}{150 \text{ mg}} \times \frac{1 \text{ ml}}{1} = 2.7 \text{ ml}$$

   Dimensional analysis method:

   $$\frac{1 \text{ ml}}{150 \text{ mg}} \times \frac{400 \text{ mg}}{1} = 2.7 \text{ ml}$$

9. *Answer:* 0.75 ml

   Ratio and proportion method:

   $$\frac{1 \text{ ml}}{2 \text{ mg}} = \frac{x \text{ ml}}{1.5 \text{ mg}} = 0.75 \text{ ml}$$

   Dosage formula method:

   $$\frac{1.5 \text{ mg}}{2.0 \text{ mg}} \times \frac{1 \text{ ml}}{1} = 0.75 \text{ ml}$$

   Dimensional analysis method:

   $$\frac{1 \text{ ml}}{2 \text{ mg}} \times \frac{1.5 \text{ mg}}{1} = 0.75 \text{ ml}$$

10. *Answer:* 1.5 tablets

    Ratio and proportion method:

    $$\frac{1 \text{ tablet}}{10 \text{ milligrams}} = \frac{x \text{ tablets}}{15 \text{ milligrams}} = 1.5 \text{ tablets}$$

    Dosage formula method:

    $$\frac{15 \text{ milligrams}}{10 \text{ milligrams}} \times \frac{1 \text{ tablet}}{1} = 1.5 \text{ tablets}$$

    Dimensional analysis method:

    $$\frac{1 \text{ tablet}}{10 \text{ milligrams}} \times \frac{15 \text{ milligrams}}{1} = 1.5 \text{ tablets}$$

11. *Answer:* 1.5 ml

    Ratio and proportion method:

    2 ml / 100 mg $\times$ x ml / 75 mg = 1.5 ml

    Dosage formula method:

    $$\frac{75 \text{ mg}}{100 \text{ mg}} \times \frac{2 \text{ ml}}{1} = 1.5 \text{ ml}$$

    Dimensional analysis method:

    $$\frac{2 \text{ ml}}{100 \text{ mg}} \times \frac{75 \text{ mg}}{1} = 1.5 \text{ ml}$$

12. *Answer:* 10 ml

    Ratio and proportion method:

    $$\frac{5 \text{ ml}}{12.5 \text{ mg}} = \frac{x \text{ ml}}{25 \text{ mg}} = 10 \text{ ml}$$

    Dosage formula method:

    $$\frac{25 \text{ mg}}{12.5 \text{ mg}} \times \frac{5 \text{ ml}}{1} = 10 \text{ ml}$$

    Dimensional analysis method:

    $$\frac{5 \text{ ml}}{12.5 \text{ mg}} \times \frac{25 \text{ mg}}{1} = 10 \text{ ml}$$

13. *Answer:* 0.15 ml

    Ratio and proportion method:

    $$\frac{1 \text{ milliliter}}{100 \text{ units}} = \frac{x \text{ milliliters}}{15 \text{ units}} = 0.15 \text{ milliliter}$$

    Dosage formula method:

    $$\frac{15 \text{ units}}{100 \text{ units}} \times \frac{1 \text{ milliliter}}{1} = 0.15 \text{ milliliter}$$

    Dimensional analysis method:

    $$\frac{1 \text{ milliliter}}{100 \text{ units}} \times \frac{15 \text{ units}}{1} = 0.15 \text{ milliliter}$$

14. *Answer:* 0.7 ml

   Ratio and proportion method:

   $$\frac{1 \text{ milliliter}}{15,000 \text{ units}} = \frac{x \text{ milliliter}}{10,000 \text{ units}} = 0.7 \text{ milliliter}$$

   Dosage formula method:

   $$\frac{10,000 \text{ units}}{15,000 \text{ units}} \times \frac{x \text{ milliliter}}{1} = 0.7 \text{ milliliter}$$

   Dimensional analysis method:

   $$\frac{1 \text{ milliliter}}{15,000 \text{ units}} \times \frac{10,000 \text{ units}}{1} = 0.7 \text{ milliliter}$$

15. *Answer:* 0.4 ml

   Ratio and proportion method:

   $$\frac{1 \text{ ml}}{5 \text{ mg}} = \frac{x \text{ ml}}{2 \text{ mg}} = 0.4 \text{ ml}$$

   Dosage formula method:

   $$\frac{2 \text{ mg}}{5 \text{ mg}} \times \frac{1 \text{ ml}}{1} = 0.4 \text{ ml}$$

   Dimensional analysis method:

   $$\frac{1 \text{ ml}}{5 \text{ mg}} \times \frac{2 \text{ mg}}{1} = 0.4 \text{ ml}$$

Reference

Potter, A. P., & Perry, A. G. (2005). *Fundamentals of nursing*. St. Louis, MO: Mosby.

3 Medication Administration Safety

Introduction

A mathematics text designed for nurses and allied health professionals would be remiss if it did not discuss safety in administering medications. Many nursing faculty and healthcare educators believe it is necessary to review this content with students in order to stress the importance of getting it right the first time. This chapter reviews the steps in safely administering medications and reviews techniques for pouring medications. Clinical scenarios are presented to demonstrate these safety measures.

The Six Steps to Safely Giving Medications

The goal for any nurse or healthcare professional is to avoid making a medication error, some of which may cause harm to the client. Nursing professionals and allied health professionals follow established guidelines to ensure the proper administration of medications. Each of the following steps is discussed individually:

- Step 1: The Right Drug
- Step 2: The Right Dose
- Step 3: The Right Route
- Step 4: The Right Time
- Step 5: The Right Client
- Step 6: The Right Documentation

Also refer to the guidelines in the following tip for preventing medication errors.

M edication Administration Tip

To aid in preventing medication administration errors, remember the following guidelines (Potter & Perry, 2005, p. 836):

- Read all labels carefully.
- Double-check large quantities of pills and liquids.
- Never guess when handwriting is illegible.
- Look up new or unfamiliar medications.
- Properly identify clients.
- Double-check all calculations.

Step 1: The Right Drug

Before pouring any medication for administration, check the drug order against the physician's order. A comparison between the written order and the medication administration record (MAR) is the best method for ensuring that the right drug is prepared for dispensing.

Also, check the label on the container three times before handing over any medication to a client.

1. The first check is completed when the medication is removed from the cart.
2. The second check is made before the dose is poured.
3. The third check is made after the drug is poured but before it is given to the client.

Other measures to ensure getting the drug right are as follows:

- Anyone who is administering medications must dispense only what he or she has poured. Never give a medication that you have not personally prepared.
- If a client has a question about the medication being correct or is hesitant about taking unfamiliar medications, always give the client the benefit of the doubt and check the drug: The client's concerns are probably valid.
- Never leave medications in a client's room or at the bedside. If the client is unable to take the medication, remove it from the room and return with it when the client can take it.

M edication Administration Tip

Intravenous injections of medications produce rapid absorption of the medication due to immediate access of the system circulation (Potter & Perry, 2005, p. 825).

Clinical Scenario

A hospitalized client rings her call bell and tells her nurse she has pain and wants a pill. The nurse checks the MAR and sees an order for Motrin 600 mg po (by mouth) q 4–6 h PRN for pain alternating with Percocet tabs 1–2 po q 4 h PRN for pain. The nurse prepares the Motrin for administration. Upon entering the room, the nurse discovers that the client is requesting a Percocet tablet, not the Motrin tablet the nurse has poured. The client requests that the nurse leave the Motrin on her nightstand while obtaining the Percocet pill. The client promises not to touch the medication until the nurse returns. The client appears alert and oriented. What should the nurse do next?

1. Respect the client's wishes and leave the Motrin while obtaining the Percocet.
2. Leave the Motrin but place it out of the client's reach.
3. Take the Motrin back to the medication room while pouring the Percocet.
4. Insist the client take the Motrin before leaving the room.

Answer

3. Never leave medication in the client's room unattended. The nurse should take the Motrin while obtaining the Percocet and then give the client the correct medication. It is also important to remember to assess exactly what medication the client is requesting before pouring any drug.

Step 2: The Right Dose

Having determined that the drug is the right one, the nurse next ensures that the correct dosage is administered. With the introduction of unit dosing in many facilities, the occurrences of dosage errors is decreasing. However, in many instances healthcare professionals must still pour drugs from multidose containers or modify the unit dose provided, increasing the chances of committing a medication administration error.

Another circumstance that increases the odds of mismedicating a client is when the nurse must mathematically calculate the correct dosage. All medication calculations should be double-checked for accuracy. If there is any reason to doubt the accuracy of the calculation, have a second nurse verify the medication dose or call on the pharmacist to assist. Never medicate when in doubt about the dosing accuracy.

Tablets that need to be broken must be scored and divided evenly. If a tablet is split unevenly, discard the entire tablet. Use a cutting device to ensure that the two halves are equal. Some experienced nurses are able to evenly split a tablet in half using gloved hands, but this practice is not recommended. Once a scored tablet is broken, rewrap the remaining half and relabel it for future use.

If a pill needs to be crushed, crush only tablets that are *not* timed-released (TR), extended-released (ER), or enteric-coated (EC). Also, use a clean pill-crushing device.

If the client is unable to take the dose as dispensed, investigate the possibility of dosing in a liquid form.

M edication Administration Tip

> When medications are taken over prolonged periods of time or when they accumulate in the blood because of impaired metabolism and/or excretion, the client may develop toxic or lethal effects (Potter & Perry, 2005, p. 829).

Clinical Scenario

A client with rheumatoid arthritis is to receive EC aspirin grain V po at 10 am. The nurse pours the medication and discovers that the client states she always takes grain X at home and wants the pills crushed and put into applesauce. She states that she does this at home all the time and has no problems. What should the nurse do next?

1. Comply with the client's request because this is what she is used to doing.
2. Insist the client take the prepared dose and swallow the tablet whole.
3. Dissolve the grain V tablet in warm water for the client to drink.
4. Contact the ordering physician to verify the dose and to obtain an order for a liquid preparation of the medication.

Answer

4. The nurse should always verify the dose when questioned by the client and remember to not crush an enteric-coated pill. It is inappropriate to insist that the client take the medication whole. Dissolving enteric-coated medications is not recommended. The nurse should call the ordering physician about a liquid medication order.

Step 3: The Right Route

Once the nurse has determined that the right dose has been obtained, the next step is to ensure that the medication is administered via the right route. For all medications ordered, nurses and allied healthcare professionals involved with medication administration must ascertain that the ordering physician or healthcare administrator has designated the route of administration. If the route is not clearly written, call the prescriber and clarify the order to include route to dispense. Also, read the label on the medication to ensure that the route for administration is listed.

M edication Administration Tip

> Prepare injections only from preparations designed for parenteral use. The injection of a liquid designed for oral use can produce local complications (Potter & Perry, 2005, p. 842).

Clinical Scenario

A client returns from the postanesthesia care unit (PACU) and is to receive Demerol 50 mg po for postoperative pain. The nurse pours one 50-mg tablet of Demerol and brings it to the client's bedside. The client states he is unable to swallow pills and requests liquid medication. The nurse returns to the narcotic box and discovers only injectable vials of Demerol. What should be the nurse's next action?

1. Administer the injectable liquid Demerol to the client by mouth.
2. Call the pharmacist to obtain an oral liquid form of Demerol.
3. Crush the Demerol pill and place it in applesauce for the postoperative client.
4. Call the physician for a new pain medication order for the client.

Answer

2. The healthcare professional administering the Demerol should contact the pharmacist to obtain a liquid form of Demerol. Injectable liquids may not be administered by mouth. Crushing the medication and giving it in applesauce after the client has requested a liquid form of the drug is inappropriate. You do not have to call the physician for a new medication order because the order is already for oral administration.

M edication Administration Tip

> Routes of medication administration include oral, sublingual (under the tongue), buccal (placed against oral mucous membranes of the cheek), topical, inhalation, and parenteral injections such as intradermal, subcutaneous, intramuscular, and intravenous (Potter & Perry, 2005, p. 829).

Step 4: The Right Time

Having determined the right route for the medication to be administered, the allied health professional next confirms that it is the right time for the medication to be given. Take special care to ensure that the institutional policy for medication times is followed. For example, a medication that is ordered every 6 hours would be given around-the-clock in four divided doses, such as 12 mn, 6 am, 12 noon, and 6 pm. A medication that is ordered QID (during the daytime) would be given four times during the client waking hours, such as 9 am, 1 pm, 5 pm, and 9 pm.

Also verify the times on the order. Healthcare providers must know exactly when the medication, such as preprocedure medication or on-call medication, is to be given. Medications that are ordered as STAT (right away) are given without delay. Some medications are ordered to be given on a PRN (when necessary) basis, and it is up to the nurse and or healthcare professional to determine the appropriateness of medicating the client at a specific time.

M edication Administration Tip

Intentional and predictable effects from medications are known as therapeutic effects (Potter & Perry, 2005, p. 829).

Clinical Scenario

A client has an order for Seconal 100 mg QHS PRN for sleep. The healthcare professional offers the client a sleeping pill at 9 pm and 10 pm. Both times the client refuses. At 3 am the client rings his call bell and requests a sleeping pill. What would be the nurse's most appropriate action?

1. Medicate the client as requested.
2. Bring the client crackers and warm milk.
3. Tell the client it is too late for sleeping medication and suggest he watch television.
4. Contact the physician on call.

Answer

4. Administering a sleeping pill at 3 am is typically considered to be too late into the night. The client has not requested crackers and milk. It is inappropriate to suggest the client watch television. The correct action is to contact the physician on call and discuss the client's needs.

Step 5: The Right Client

With the correct time for medication administration ascertained, the healthcare provider determines that the right client is receiving the medication. To verify a client's correct identity:

- First compare the client name on the medication administration record (MAR) to the client's name on his or her identification bracelet.
- Next, ask the client to state his or her name. If a client protests, simply explain that the procedure for correctly identifying clients is routine.

This is also the time to check the client's allergy bracelet to determine whether there are any known medication allergies. If the client's identification bracelet is illegible or missing, have a colleague familiar with the client identify the client and then reband the client's wrist.

M edication Administration Tip

Unintended but predictable effects from medications are known as side effects (Potter & Perry, 2005, p. 829).

Clinical Scenario

A newly graduated nurse is administering medications. Upon entering the room of an elderly client, the nurse asks the client whether she is Mrs. Robbins. The client answers "Yes," and the nurse prepares to administer medications. The nursing supervisor enters the room and greets the client by saying, "Good morning, Mrs. Avery." What should be the newly graduated nurse's immediate response?

1. Ask the client if she is Mrs. Avery.
2. Tell the nursing supervisor that the client's name is Mrs. Robbins.
3. Withhold the medications until the client's identity is certain.
4. Administer the medications as planned, and speak to the supervisor afterward in private.

Answer

3. Medications should not be administered until the client's identity is certain. When asking a client to state his or her name, do not include the client's name in the question. It is also imperative to check the identification band on the client's wrist after the name is verified. Correcting the nursing supervisor is inappropriate and administering the medication at this time would be unsafe.

M edication Administration Tip

> Always check the client's identification bracelet.

Step 6: The Right Documentation

Once the client is correctly and positively identitified, the final step is completing the right documentation. This sixth step is included to increase the safety standards regarding medication administration for clients. Right documentation is a two-part responsibility for the healthcare professional administering medications.

1. First, making the right entry for the medication on the medical administration record is imperative. The entry must include the client's name, allergies, and medication name, dose, route, and time.
2. After the medication is administered, the healthcare professional has to accurately document the drug given. This documentation should include the drug name, dose, route, and time. Complete this documentation immediately *after* administering the medication, never before.

M edication Administration Tip

> The nurse's six rights for safe medication administration are (Cook, 1999, p. 8):
>
> 1. The right to a complete and clearly written order.
> 2. The right to have the correct drug route and dose dispensed.
> 3. The right to have access to information.
> 4. The right to have policies on medication administration.
> 5. The right to administer medications safely and to identify problems in the system.
> 6. The right to stop, think, and be vigilant when administering medications.

M edication Administration Tip

Regarding the administration of medication, a client has the right (Potter & Perry, 2005, p. 843):

1. To be informed of the medication's name, purpose, action, and potential undesired effects.
2. To refuse a medication, regardless of the consequences.
3. To have qualified nurses or physicians assess a medication history, including allergies.
4. To be properly advised of the experimental nature of medication therapy and to give written consent for its use.
5. To receive labeled medications safely without discomfort in accordance with the six rights of medication administration.
6. To receive appropriate supportive therapy in relation to medication therapy.
7. To not receive unnecessary medications.

M edication Administration Tip

Here are some tips on how to prepare oral medications correctly and safely:

- Prepare to administer oral medications for one client at a time. Never pour medications for multiple clients at the same time. Doing so may lead to confusion and medication errors.
- After clarifying the medication order on the MAR, remove the medication from the unit's stock supply or from the unit's dose drawer. When you do so, read the medication label completely.
- Once you have removed the medication from the drawer, read the label a second time, and also check the expiration date and complete any necessary calculations.
- Before actually pouring the medication, compare it to the MAR and assess the client's drug allergy history.
- Now it's time to pour the medication.
- Once the oral medication has been poured, read the label a third time, and compare it to the MAR before discarding it. These three safety checks are important measures to correctly and safely administer oral medications.

Mathematical Word Problems

In addition to observing client's rights and learning proper techniques to administer medications safely, anyone who administers medications must know how to solve mathematical word problems, which are typically used in determining competence in giving medications. Here are some simple steps to follow in determining the correct drugs, dose, route, and time from mathematical word problems:

- *Read the word problem carefully.* This advice may sound rudimentary, but the importance of this step cannot be overemphasized. Reading carefully means to understand *exactly* what the problem is asking. Pay attention to words that stand out, such as words that are *italicized*, **bolded**, or <u>underlined</u>. These words are meant to guide you in determining the correct answer.

- *Know what to include in your calculations and what to omit.* Very often mathematical word problems contain extraneous data that are intended to distract. When assigning significance to information in word problems, remember that you need certain pieces of data, such as

  - what drug/medication is ordered;
  - how much is required (dose);
  - how much is supplied; and
  - how it is supplied (route).

- *Make sure your answer is reasonable.* In other words, giving 1 or 2 tablets to a client is reasonable, but giving 20 tablets is not. Giving 1 to 3 ml of fluid by intramuscular injection is reasonable, but giving a 60-ml intramuscular injection is not. When you have completed your calculations, ask yourself whether the answer requires you to give a dose that makes sense.

- *Double-check your answer.* Beginning students in grammar school learn this technique. You may use any procedure that you are comfortable with. Typically, either the ratio and proportion method, dosage formula method, or dimensional analysis method ensures an accurate assessment of your answer (see Chapter 2). If ever you are in doubt about your calculations, have a colleague, pharmacist, or physician check them. There is no shame in asking for help. There is potential tragedy in failing to do so.

Example Mathematical Word Problems

See how the following mathematical word problems are solved. Refer to the six steps as needed. Remember to show all work and proof all answers.

1. *Ordered:* Folic acid 1 mg po in liquid form every morning for a client weighing 115 lb
   Supply: 50-ml bottle of folic acid 1 mg per 5 ml
   Give: _____
   Solve and double-check:
   Ratio and proportion method:

   $$\frac{1\,mg}{5\,ml} = \frac{1\,mg}{x\,ml} = 5\,ml$$

   Dosage formula method:

   $$\frac{1\,mg}{1\,mg} \times 5\,ml = 5\,ml$$

   Dimensional analysis method:

   $$x\,ml = \frac{5\,ml}{1\,mg} \times \frac{1\,mg}{1} = 5\,ml$$

   Answer: 5 ml
   What data can you omit? You most probably may omit the client's weight and the size of the bottle. This information may be important for other reasons, but it is not needed to solve the calculation issue.
   Is your answer reasonable? Yes. It is reasonable to give 5 ml po.

2. *Ordered:* NPH insulin 23 units subcutaneous every morning for a client with diabetes mellitus
   Supply: 10-ml vial NPH insulin 100 units per 1 ml
   Give: _____

Solve and double-check:

    Ratio and proportion method:

$$\frac{100\ \text{units}}{1\ \text{milliliter}} = \frac{23\ \text{units}}{x\ \text{milliliter}} = 0.23\ \text{milliliter}$$

    Dosage formula method:

$$\frac{23\ \text{units}}{100\ \text{units}} \times \frac{1\ \text{milliliter}}{1} = 0.23\ \text{milliliter}$$

    Dimensional analysis method:

$$x\ \text{ml} = \frac{1\ \text{milliliter}}{100\ \text{units}} \times \frac{23\ \text{units}}{1} = 0.23\ \text{milliliter}$$

Answer: 0.23 milliliter
What data can you omit? The client's diagnosis and the size of the vial are important pieces of information but not needed to solve this equation.
Is your answer reasonable? Yes. It is reasonable to give 0.23 milliliter subcutaneously.

3. *Ordered:* Keflex 1 gram po QID for a client with pneumonia. The client is allergic to penicillin (PCN) and has taken Keflex in the past without incident.
   Supply: Keflex 500-mg scored tablets
   Give: _____
   Solve and double-check: First you must change 1 gram into milligrams (1 gram = 1000 milligrams).

       Ratio and proportion method:

   $$\frac{500\ \text{milligrams}}{1\ \text{tablet}} = \frac{1000\ \text{milligrams}}{x\ \text{tablets}} = 2\ \text{tablets}$$

       Dosage formula method:

   $$\frac{1\ \text{gram}}{500\ \text{milligrams}} \times \frac{1\ \text{tablet}}{1}$$

   $$\frac{1000\ \text{milligrams}}{500\ \text{milligrams}} \times \frac{1\ \text{tablet}}{1} = 2\ \text{tablets}$$

       Dimensional analysis method:

   $$x\ \text{tablets} = \frac{1\ \text{tablet}}{500\ \text{milligrams}} \times \frac{1000\ \text{milligrams}}{1} = 2\ \text{tablets}$$

Answer: 2 tablets
What data can you omit? The client's diagnosis and the dosing frequency are useful information but not needed for the solution to this problem.
Is your answer reasonable? Yes. It is reasonable to give a client 2 tablets.

Practice Mathematical Word Problems

Now solve and double-check the following mathematical word problems on your own, using the dosage formula, the ratio and proportion, and the dimensional analysis methods. The answers to the questions are at the end of this chapter. Remember to show all work and to proof all answers.

1. *Ordered:* Synthroid 0.075-milligram po every morning for a client with hypothyroidism
   Supply: Synthroid 0.15-milligram scored tablets
   Give: _____

Ratio and proportion method:

Dosage formula method:

Dimensional analysis method:

What data can you omit?

Is your answer reasonable?

2. *Ordered:* Penicillin G 150,000 units intramuscularly Q8H for a postoperative client × 4 doses
   Supply: Penicillin G 1,000,000 units in 20 milliliters of reconstituted solution
   Give: _____
   Ratio and proportion method:

   Dosage formula method:

   Dimensional analysis method:

   What data can you omit?

   Is your answer reasonable?

3. *Ordered:* Chloral hydrate grain VII$\overline{ss}$ as a one-time dose for a preoperative client. The client states he is anxious about surgery in the morning.
   Supply: Chloral hydrate 0.25-gram tablets
   Give: _____
   Ratio and proportion method:

   Dosage formula method:

   Dimensional analysis method:

   What data can you omit?

   Is your answer reasonable?

4. *Ordered:* Morphine gr $^1/_{200}$ IM Q4h PRN for severe pain for a client who states her pain scale is a 9
   Supply: Morphine 0.4 mg in 1-ml single-dose ampules
   Give: _____
   Ratio and proportion method:

   Dosage formula method:

   Dimensional analysis method:

   What data can you omit?

   Is your answer reasonable?

5. *Ordered:* Atropine 0.5 mg IM on call to the operating room for a client who weighs 200 lb (91 kg)
   Supply: Atropine grain 1/150 per ml in a 5-ml vial
   Give: _____
   Ratio and proportion method:

   Dosage formula method:

   Dimensional analysis method:

   What data can you omit?

   Is your answer reasonable?

POSTTEST

1. List the guidelines useful in preventing medication administration errors.
2. Describe the six rights of medication administration.
3. Identify the nurse's six rights for safe medication administration.
4. List the client's rights regarding the administration of medication.
5. Discuss the steps to be followed in ensuring client safety when reading mathematical word problems.

Answers

Answers to Practice Mathematical Word Problems

1. *Answer:* ½ tablet
   Solve and double-check:

   Ratio and proportion method:

   $$\frac{0.15 \text{ milligram}}{1 \text{ tablet}} = \frac{0.075 \text{ milligram}}{x \text{ tablets}} = \text{½ tablet}$$

   Dosage formula method:

   $$\frac{0.075 \text{ milligram}}{0.15 \text{ milligram}} \times \frac{1 \text{ scored tablet}}{1} = \text{½ tablet}$$

   Dimensional analysis method:

   $$x \text{ tablets} = \frac{1 \text{ tablet}}{0.15 \text{ milligram}} \times \frac{0.75 \text{ milligram}}{1} = \text{½ tablet}$$

   What data can you omit? The client's diagnosis is not needed to solve the equation.
   Is your answer reasonable? Yes. It is reasonable to give a client ½ tablet.

2. *Answer:* 3 milliliters
   Solve and double-check:

   Ratio and proportion method:

   $$\frac{1,000,000 \text{ units}}{20 \text{ milliliters}} = \frac{150,000 \text{ units}}{x \text{ milliliters}} = 3 \text{ milliliters}$$

   Dosage formula method:

   $$\frac{150,000 \text{ units}}{1,000,000 \text{ units}} \times \frac{20 \text{ milliliters}}{1} = 3 \text{ milliliters}$$

Dimensional analysis method:

$$x \text{ ml} = \frac{20 \text{ milliliters}}{1,000,000 \text{ units}} \times \frac{150,000 \text{ units}}{1} = 3 \text{ milliliters}$$

What data can you omit? The postoperative status of the client and the number of doses are not relevant to the equation.
Is your answer reasonable? Yes. It is reasonable to give a client a 3-milliliter injection.

3. *Answer:* 2 tablets
   Solve and double-check: First you must change grain VII$\overline{ss}$ into grams (grain VII$\overline{ss}$ = 0.5 gram).
   Ratio and proportion method:

   $$\frac{0.25 \text{ gram}}{1 \text{ tablet}} = \frac{0.5 \text{ gram}}{x \text{ tablets}} = 2 \text{ tablets}$$

   Dosage formula method:

   $$\frac{0.5 \text{ gram}}{0.25 \text{ gram}} \times \frac{1 \text{ tablet}}{1} = 2 \text{ tablets}$$

   Dimensional analysis method:

   $$x \text{ tablets} = \frac{1 \text{ tablet}}{0.25 \text{ gram}} \times \frac{0.5 \text{ gram}}{1} = 2 \text{ tablets}$$

What data can you omit? Knowing your client is preoperative and anxious is an important factor in his care but not necessary for this problem.
Is your answer reasonable? Yes. It is reasonable to give a client 2 tablets.

4. *Answer:* 0.75 ml
   Solve and double-check: First you must convert gr $^{1}/_{200}$ to mg (gr $^{1}/_{200}$ = 0.3 mg).
   Ratio and proportion method:

   $$\frac{0.4 \text{ mg}}{1 \text{ ml}} = \frac{0.3 \text{ mg}}{x \text{ ml}} = 0.75 \text{ ml}$$

   Dosage formula method:

   $$\frac{0.3 \text{ mg}}{0.4 \text{ mg}} \times \frac{1 \text{ ml}}{1} = 0.75 \text{ ml}$$

   Dimensional analysis method:

   $$x \text{ ml} = \frac{1 \text{ ml}}{0.4 \text{ mg}} \times \frac{0.3 \text{ mg}}{1} = 0.75 \text{ ml}$$

What data can you omit? It is important to know that the client's pain is severe and warrants the morphine injection, but this fact does not enter into the calculation.
Is your answer reasonable? Yes. It is reasonable to give an injection of 0.75 ml.

5. *Answer:* 1.25 ml
   Solve and double-check: First you must convert gr $^{1}/_{150}$ to mg (gr $^{1}/_{150}$ = 0.4 mg).
   Ratio and proportion method:

   $$\frac{0.4 \text{ mg}}{1 \text{ ml}} = \frac{0.5 \text{ mg}}{x \text{ ml}} = 1.25 \text{ ml}$$

Dosage formula method:

$$\frac{0.5\,\text{mg}}{0.4\,\text{mg}} \times \frac{1\,\text{ml}}{1} = 1.25\,\text{ml}$$

Dimensional analysis method:

$$x\,\text{ml} = \frac{1\,\text{ml}}{0.4\,\text{mg}} \times \frac{0.5\,\text{mg}}{1} = 1.25\,\text{ml}$$

What data can you omit? The client's weight is irrelevant. Also, knowing the vial was 5 ml hopefully did not fool you into using that information in the calculation.

Is your answer reasonable? Yes. It is reasonable to administer a 1.25-ml injection.

Answers to Posttest

1. The guidelines useful in preventing medication administration errors are as follows:

   - Read all labels carefully.
   - Double-check large quantities of pills and liquids.
   - Never guess when handwriting is illegible.
   - Look up new or unfamiliar medications.
   - Properly identify clients.
   - Double-check all calculations.

2. The six rights of medication administration are as follows:

   - The right drug—trade/generic name the same as physician order
   - The right dose—the exact amount ordered by healthcare attendant
   - The right route—oral, IM, IV, subcu, topical, buccal, transdermal, intradermal
   - The right time—PRN meds on time; standard meds 1 hr before to 1 hr after
   - The right client—check ID band, compare to MAR, and have client state name
   - The right documentation—med and response to med after administration

3. The nurse's six rights for safe medication administration are as follows:

   - The right to a complete and clearly written order.
   - The right to have the correct drug route and dose dispensed.
   - The right to have access to information.
   - The right to have policies on medication administration.
   - The right to administer medications safely and to identify problems in the system.
   - The right to stop, think, and be vigilant when administering medications.

4. The client's rights regarding medication administration are as follows:

   - To be informed of the medication's name, purpose, action, and potential undesired effects.
   - To refuse a medication, regardless of the consequences.
   - To have qualified nurses or physicians assess a medication history, including allergies.
   - To be properly advised of the experimental nature of medication therapy and to give written consent for its use.

- To receive labeled medications safely without discomfort in accordance with the six rights of medication administration.
- To receive appropriate supportive therapy in relation to medication therapy.
- To not receive unnecessary medications.

5. The steps to be followed in ensuring client safety when reading mathematical word problems are as follows:

- *Read the word problem carefully.* This advice may sound rudimentary, but the importance of this step cannot be overemphasized. Reading carefully means to understand *exactly* what the problem is asking. Pay attention to words that stand out, such as words that are *italicized*, **bolded**, or <u>underlined</u>. These words are meant to guide you in determining the correct answer.

- *Know what to include in your calculations and what to omit.* Very often mathematical word problems contain extraneous data that are intended to distract. When assigning significance to information in word problems, remember that you need certain pieces of data, such as

  - what drug/medication is ordered;
  - how much is required (dose);
  - how much is supplied; and
  - how it is supplied (route).

- *Make sure your answer is reasonable.* In other words, giving 1 or 2 tablets to a client is reasonable, but giving 20 tablets is not. Giving 1 to 3 ml of fluid by intramuscular injection is reasonable, but giving a 60-ml intramuscular injection is not. When you have completed your calculations, ask yourself whether the answer requires you to give a dose that makes sense.

- *Double-check your answer.* Beginning students in grammar school learn this technique. You may use any procedure that you are comfortable with. Typically, either the ratio and proportion method, dosage formula method, or dimensional analysis method ensures an accurate assessment of your answer (see Chapter 2). If ever you are in doubt about your calculations, have a colleague, pharmacist, or physician check them. There is no shame in asking for help. There is potential tragedy in failing to do so.

References

Cook, M. C. (1999). Nurses' six rights for safe medication administration. *Massachusetts Nurse, 69*(6), 8.

Potter, A. P., & Perry, A. G. (2005). *Fundamentals of nursing.* St. Louis, MO: Mosby.

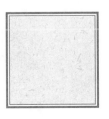

4 Identifying Labels, Syringes, and Intravenous Bags

Introduction

Nurses and allied health professionals who administer medications must be able to identify the information on medication labels, syringes, and intravenous solution bags accurately and precisely. To ensure the safety of clients, this is an important skill to master before administering medication.

This chapter reviews the techniques necessary to read labels, syringes, and intravenous bags competently. Specifically, it is designed to assist you in learning how to:

- Read medication labels to obtain pertinent information and identify various intravenous solutions.
- Read a syringe.
- Select the correct size needle and syringe.
- Reconstitute powdered medications.
- Add medication to an intravenous bag of fluid.
- Draw up two types of insulin in the same syringe.

This chapter also presents examples of medication labels and intravenous labels, as well as types and sizes of syringes and needles.

Reading Medication Labels

The brand name of a medication (also known as the trade or proprietary name) is usually written in big letters on the medication label. The brand name is typically assigned by the manufacturer of the medication and has a registered mark (®) attached to it. The generic name of a medication may be written in smaller letters, placed in parentheses, or written in italics. The generic name must be included on the label to enable the filling pharmacist to dispense the generic versions as substitutes for the brand-name drugs. A brand medication is often filled with generic substitutions unless the ordering physician checks off or writes "dispense as written." See Figure 4-1.

FIGURE 4-1 Locating the brand name and generic name on a drug label.

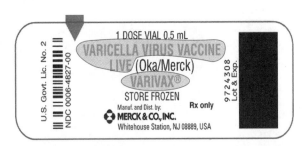

Source: Courtesy of Merck & Co., Inc.

FIGURE 4-1   (*Continued*)

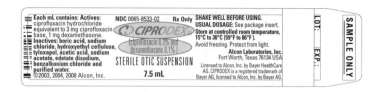

Source: © Alcon Laboratories, Inc.
Used with permission.

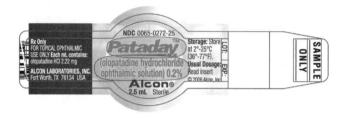

Source: © Alcon Laboratories, Inc.
Used with permission.

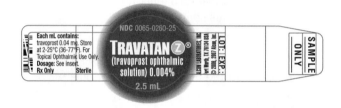

Source: © Alcon Laboratories, Inc.
Used with permission.

Source: © Alcon Laboratories, Inc.
Used with permission.

---

*M*edication Administration Tip

Varicella virus vaccine live (Varivax) is a live attenuated virus used to produce active immunity to the varicella virus, which causes chicken pox.

---

*M*edication Administration Tip

Ciprodex (ciprofloxacin) is an antibacterial agent used to treat infections caused by susceptible gram-negative bacteria.

---

*M*edication Administration Tip

Pataday/Patanol (olopatadine hydrochloride) is an antihistamine used to relieve itching caused by conjunctivitis.

---

*M*edication Administration Tip

Travatan (travoprost) is an ophthalmic solution used in the treatment of glaucoma and ocular hypertension.

Also on the medication label are (see Figure 4-2):

- The dosage strength, always included, indicating how much drug is provided in the medication container.
- The drug form, such as tablets, capsules, powders, milliliters, drops, ounces, and so on.
- The amount of the drug in the bottle or the container volume, such as the number of tablets or milliliters.

FIGURE 4-2 Locating the drug strength, drug form, and amount of the drug on a label.

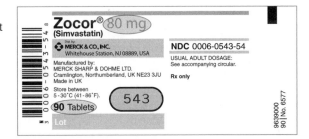

Source: Courtesy of Merck & Co., Inc.

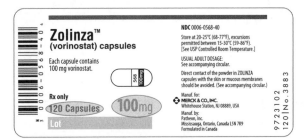

Source: Courtesy of Merck & Co., Inc.

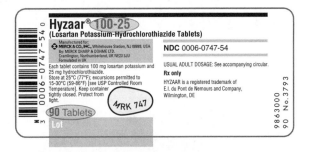

Source: Courtesy of Merck & Co., Inc.

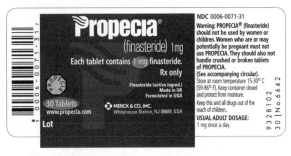

Source: Courtesy of Merck & Co., Inc.

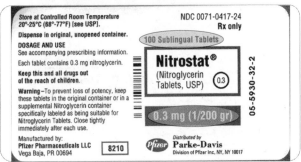

Source: © Pfizer Inc. Used with permission.

M edication Administration Tip

> Zocor (simvastatin) is an antihyperlipidemic used in the treatment of elevated total cholesterol.

M edication Administration Tip

> Zolinza (vorinostat) is a histone deacetylase (HDAC) inhibitor used in the treatment of T-cell lymphoma.

M edication Administration Tip

> Hyzaar (losartan potassium-hydrochlorothiazide) is an antihypertensive used in the treatment of elevated blood pressure.

M edication Administration Tip

> Propecia (finasteride) is an androgen hormone inhibitor used in the treatment of symptomatic benign prostatic hyperplasia (BPH).

M edication Administration Tip

> Nitrostat (Nitroglycerin) is an antianginal agent used in the treatment of acute angina.

Then look for (see Figure 4-3):

• The supply dosage, which is the number of units per specified quantity.
• Whether the container is a single or unit dose or includes multiple dosages.
• The route of administration or method of delivering the medication, such as oral, IV, IM, sublingual, topical, etc.
• Specific directions, such as the protocol for reconstituting powder, which are clearly written.

FIGURE 4-3 Locating the supply dosage, the number of doses, the route of medication administration, and specific instructions on a drug label.

Source: © Pfizer Inc. Used with permission.

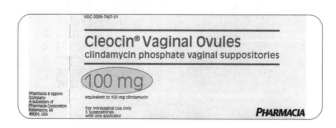

FIGURE 4-3   (*Continued*)

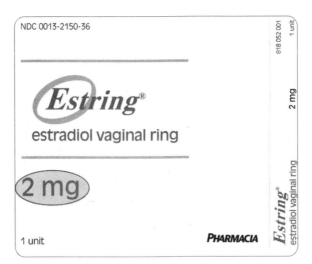

Source: © Pfizer Inc. Used with permission.

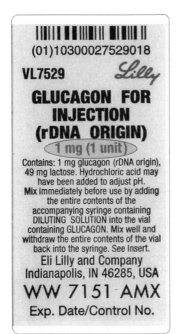

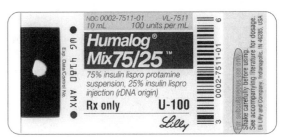

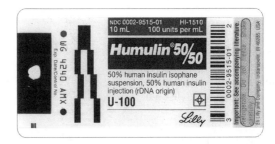

Source: © Eli Lilly and Company. Used with permission.

M edication Administration Tip

Cleocin Vaginal Ovules (clindamycin phosphate) is an antibiotic used in the treatment of bacterial vaginosis.

M edication Administration Tip

Estring (estradiol vaginal ring) is a hormone (estrogen) used in the treatment of atrophic vaginitis and the prevention of postmenopausal osteoporosis.

M edication Administration Tip

Glucagon for Injection (rDNA origin) is a glucose-elevating agent used in the treatment of hypoglycemia.

M *edication Administration Tip*

> Humalog Mix 75/25 is an antidiabetic agent (hormone insulin) used in the treatment of diabetes mellitus type 1.

M *edication Administration Tip*

> Humulin 50/50 is an antidiabetic agent (hormone insulin) used in the treatment of diabetes mellitus type 1.

Other important information found on medication labels is (see Figure 4-4):

- The drug's expiration date.
- Warnings and alerts associated with the drug, such as allergies, storage instructions, whether to shake well or do not shake, and whether to expose the medication to sunlight.
- The manufacturer's name with control or lot numbers (used mostly for drug recalls).
- The manufacturer's bar code (very important for unit dosing). The bar code, once scanned at the client's bedside before the medication is given to a client, is a check that the drug and dose are correct and documentation of that fact. See Figure 4-5.

FIGURE 4-4 Locating the expiration date, a warning or alert, storage instructions, the manufacturer's name, the lot number, and a bar code on a drug label.

Source: © Pfizer Inc. Used with permission.

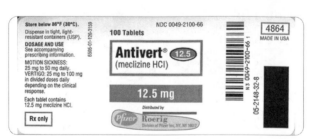

Source: © Pfizer Inc. Used with permission.

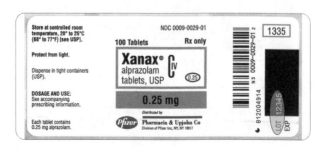

Source: © Pfizer Inc. Used with permission.

FIGURE 4-4 (*Continued*)

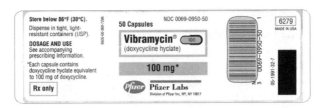

Source: © Pfizer Inc. Used with permission.

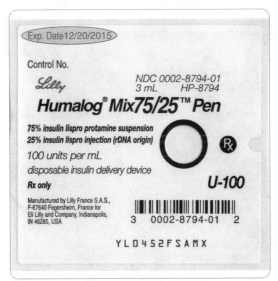

Source: © Eli Lilly and Company. Used with permission.

M edication Administration Tip

Accupril (quinapril HCL) is an antihypertensive agent used in the treatment of hypertension.

M edication Administration Tip

Antivert (meclizine HCL) is an antiemetic/anti-motion sickness agent used in the prevention and treatment of nausea, vomiting, and motion sickness.

M edication Administration Tip

Xanax (alprazolam) is an antianxiety drug used in the treatment and management of anxiety disorders.

M edication Administration Tip

Vibramycin (doxycycline hyclate) is an antibiotic used in the treatment of sensitive bacteria, particularly when Penicillin is contraindicated.

M edication Administration Tip

Humalog Mix 75/25 Pen is an antidiabetic agent (hormone insulin) in pen/unit dosing form, used in the treatment of diabetes mellitus type 1.

FIGURE 4-5   Scanning the bar code on medication ensures that the drug and dose are correct.

Source: © Simon Jarratt/Corbis/age fotostock

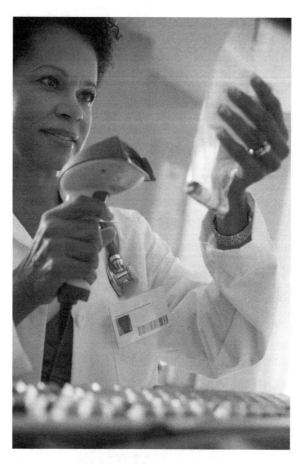

Practice Questions for Reading Medication Labels

Circle the following on the labels provided.

1. Brand name of the medication

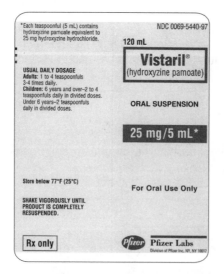

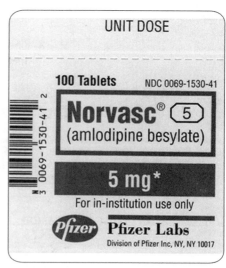

Source: © Pfizer Inc. Used with permission.

M edication Administration Tip

Vistaril (hydroxyzine pamoate) is an antianxiety/antihistamine/antiemetic used in the treatment of anxiety/pruritis/nausea and vomiting.

M *edication Administration Tip*

Norvasc (amlodipine besylate) is an antianginal/antihypertensive used in the treatment of anxiety and hypertension.

2. Trade name of the medication

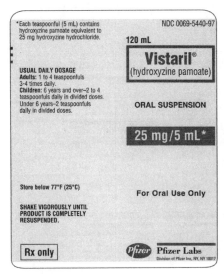 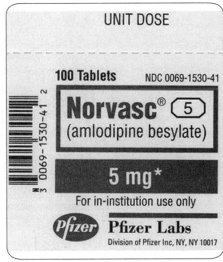

Source: © Pfizer Inc. Used with permission.

3. Generic name of the medication

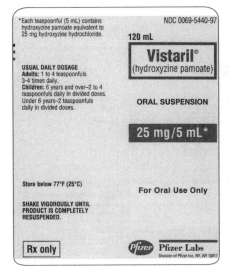 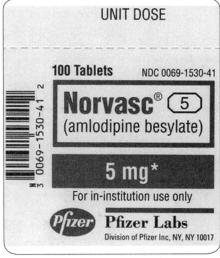

Source: © Pfizer Inc. Used with permission.

4. Drug strength

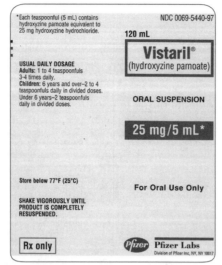 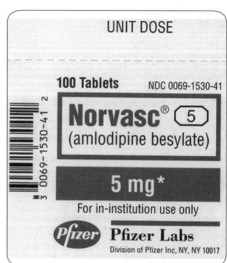

Source: © Pfizer Inc. Used with permission.

5. Drug form

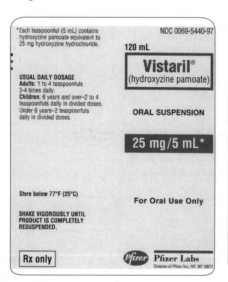 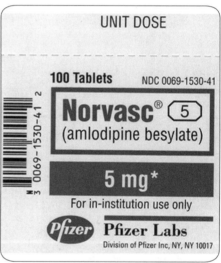

Source: © Pfizer Inc. Used with permission.

6. Drug amount

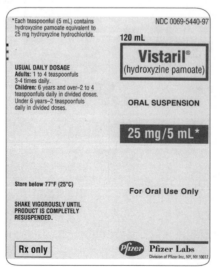 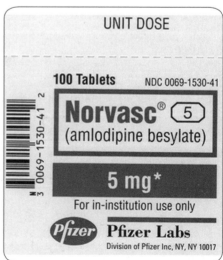

Source: © Pfizer Inc. Used with permission.

7. Supply dosage

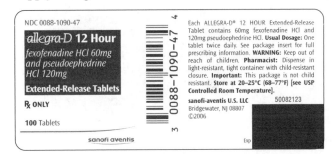

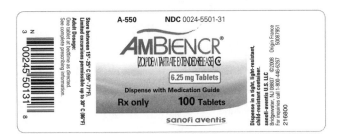

M *edication Administration Tip*

> Allegra-D 12 Hour (fexofenadine HCL and pseudoephedrine HCL) is a decongestant and antihistamine used in the treatment of symptomatic allergies.

M *edication Administration Tip*

> Ambien CR (zolpidem) is a sedative/hypnotic used in the treatment of short-term insomnia.

8. Number of dosages

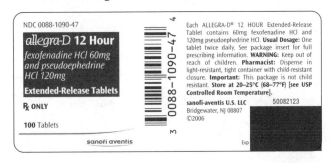

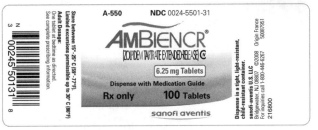

9. Route of medication

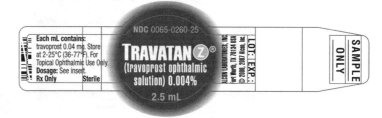

Source: © Alcon Laboratories, Inc. Used with permission.

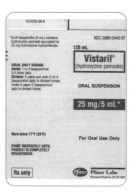

Source: © Pfizer Inc. Used with permission.

10. Expiration date

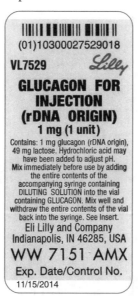

Source: © Eli Lilly and Company. Used with permission.

Source: © Alcon Laboratories, Inc. Used with permission.

11. Drug warning, alert, allergy

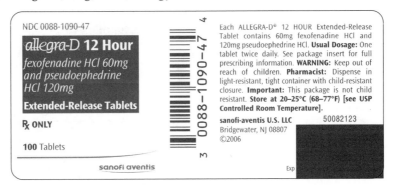

Source: © sanofi-aventis US. Used with permission.

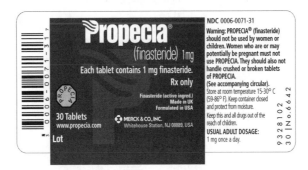

Source: Courtesy of Merck & Co., Inc.

12. Storage instructions

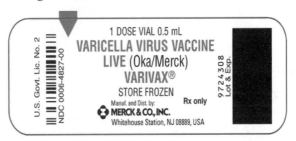

Source: Courtesy of Merck & Co., Inc.

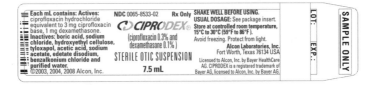

Source: © Alcon Laboratories, Inc. Used with permission.

13. Manufacturer's name

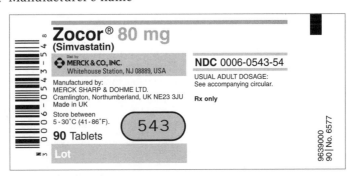

Source: Courtesy of Merck & Co., Inc.

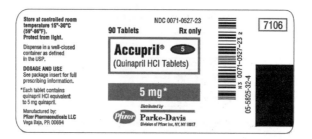

Source: © Pfizer Inc. Used with permission.

14. Lot number

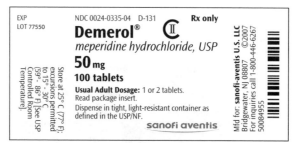

Source: © sanofi-aventis US. Used with permission.

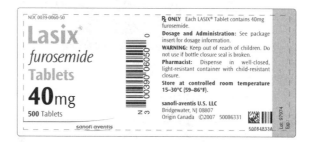

Source: © sanofi-aventis US. Used with permission.

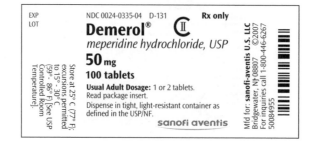

M *edication Administration Tip*

Demerol (meperidine hydrochloride) is an opioid agonist analgesic used in the treatment of moderate-to-severe acute pain.

M *edication Administration Tip*

Lasix (furosemide) is a loop diuretic used in the treatment of edema and hypertension.

15. Bar code

Source: © sanofi-aventis US. Used with permission.

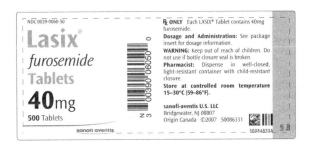

Source: © sanofi-aventis US. Used with permission.

Reading Injection Syringes

Reading injection syringes is relatively simple once you know what to look for. The following illustrations are examples of injection syringes with their various parts labeled. See Figure 4-6.

- The plunger is inside the barrel and is used to push the medication out of the syringe into tissue.
- The barrel is what holds the solution.
- The tip is where the needle attaches.

FIGURE 4-6   Three different sizes of injection syringes with parts labeled.

Source: © jkitan/Shutterstock, Inc.

Source: © AbleStock

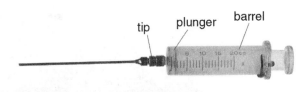

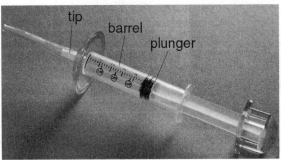

Source: © Photodisc

Insulin syringes are typically standardized to measure units. The customary calibration is 100 units (U) per 1 milliliter (ml). In other words, 1 milliliter equates to 100 units of insulin. The syringe in Figure 4-7 is a U100 insulin syringe.

FIGURE 4-7   A U100 insulin syringe.

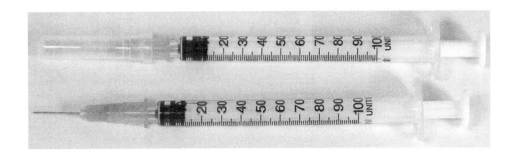

Source: © Elena Kalistratova/ Shutterstock, Inc.

A tuberculin syringe is calibrated in minims (m) and milliliters. Remember that 16 minims are equal to 1 milliliter of fluid. See Figure 4-8.

*M*edication Administration Tip

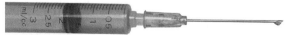

Remember that a minim is a measurement of weight that is equivalent to a drop and is abbreviated as "m." The meter is a measurement of length that is equal to 39.37 inches and abbreviated as "m" or "M."

FIGURE 4-8   A tuberculin syringe.

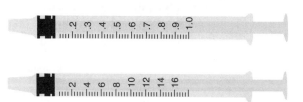

Standard syringes are calibrated in milliliters on one side and in minims on the other side. Standard syringes generally come in 3-, 5-, and 10-milliliter sizes. See Figure 4-9.

Source: © ajt/Shutterstock, Inc.

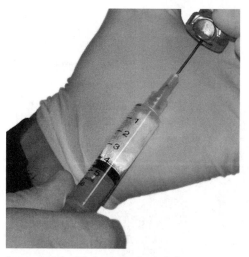

Source: © Michael G. Smith/Shutterstock, Inc.

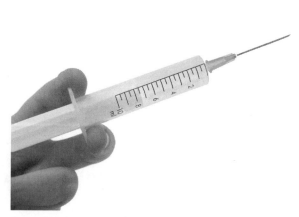

Source: © Tatiana Popova/Shutterstock, Inc.

FIGURE 4-9   Standard syringes in 3-, 5-, and 10-milliliter sizes.

Practice Questions for Reading Injection Syringes

Questions 1–3: Identify the number of units shaded in the insulin syringe:

1. _____ units

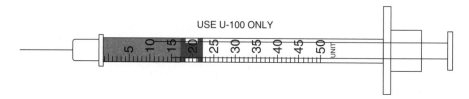

2. _____ units

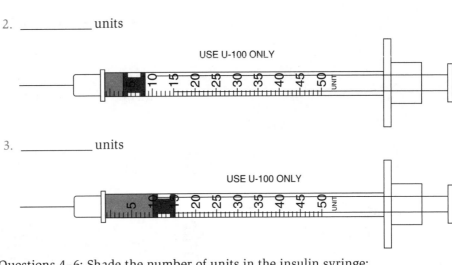

3. _____ units

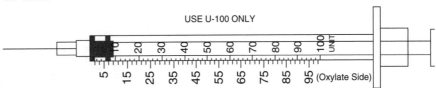

Questions 4–6: Shade the number of units in the insulin syringe:

4. 23 units

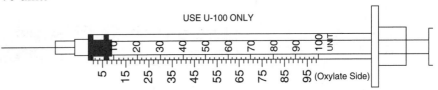

5. 70 units

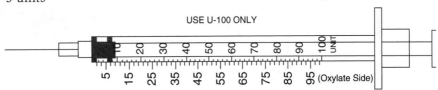

6. 5 units

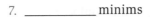
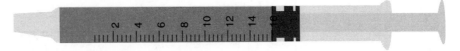

Questions 7–9: Identify the number of minims shaded in the following tuberculin syringe:

7. _____ minims

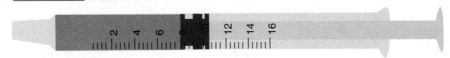

8. _____ minims

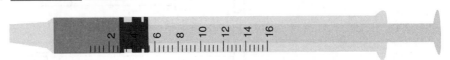

9. _____ minims

Questions 10–12: Shade the number of minims in the tuberculin syringe:

10. 12 minims

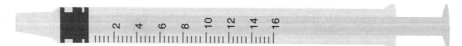

11. 5 minims

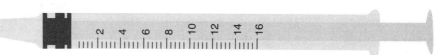

12. 2 minims

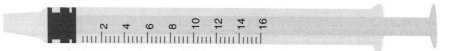

Questions 13–16: Identify the number of milliliters shaded in the standard syringe:

13. _____ milliliters

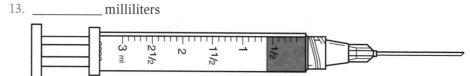

14. _____ milliliters

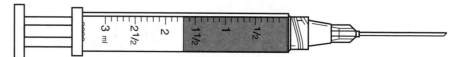

15. _____ milliliters

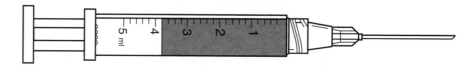

16. _____ milliliters

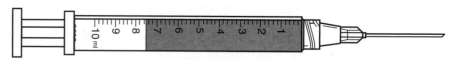

Questions 17–20: Shade in the number of milliliters in the standard syringe:

17. 1 milliliter

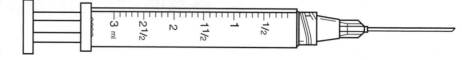

18. 1.2 ml

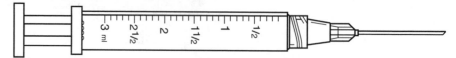

19. 2.4 ml

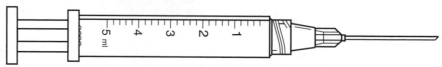

20. 6.4 ml

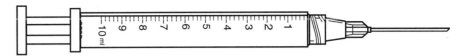

Selecting the Correct Size Needle and Syringe

Use the smallest syringe possible when giving injections. Adequate sizes are

- 1-milliliter syringes for subcutaneous injections.
- 3-milliliter syringes for intramuscular injections.

M edication Administration Tip

The ventrogluteal site is the preferred site for most injections for the adult client. The vastus lateralis is commonly used in small children and infants. The deltoid muscle is easily accessible but can be underdeveloped in many adults and is seldom used in pediatrics (Potter & Perry, 2005, p. 888). See Figure 4-10.

FIGURE 4-10   Intramuscular injection sites: ventrogluteal, vastus lateralis, and deltoid.

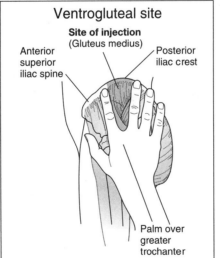

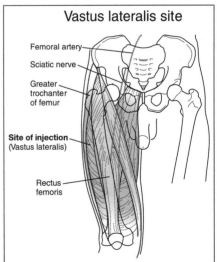

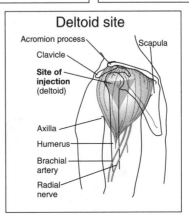

In addition to choosing the appropriate needle size, correctly identifying the parts of a needle is very important when administering an injection. See Figure 4-11.

FIGURE 4-11
Identifying the parts
of a needle.

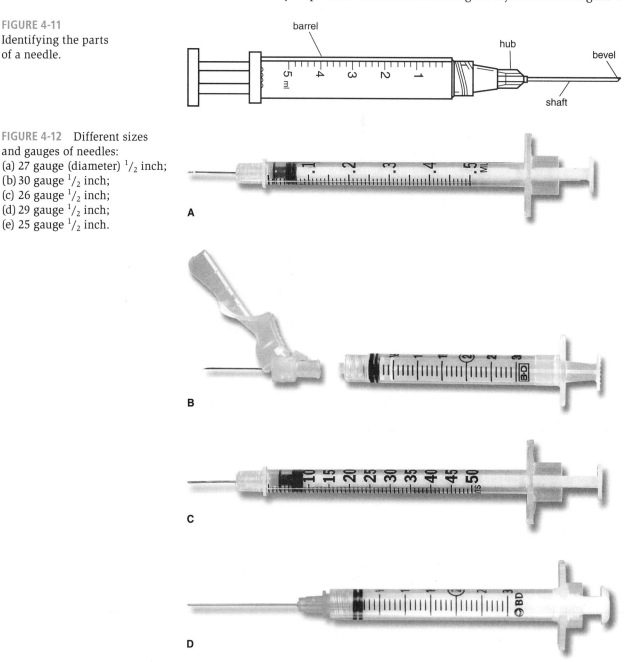

FIGURE 4-12   Different sizes
and gauges of needles:
(a) 27 gauge (diameter) $1/2$ inch;
(b) 30 gauge $1/2$ inch;
(c) 26 gauge $1/2$ inch;
(d) 29 gauge $1/2$ inch;
(e) 25 gauge $1/2$ inch.

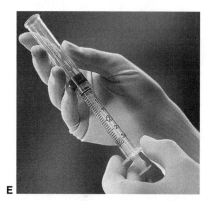

Source: Courtesy and © Becton, Dickinson
and Company.

Injectable syringes have many new safety features such as the safety sheath, which allows the nurse to cover the used needle safely and not run the risk of a fingerstick. Safety syringes come in most sizes. See Figure 4-13.

FIGURE 4-13 Safety syringes have a sheath, which allows the nurse to cover the used needle safely to avoid a fingerstick.

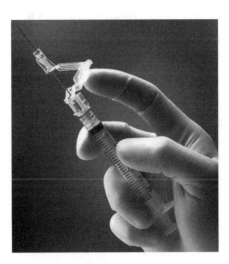

Source: Courtesy and © Becton, Dickinson and Company.

M edication Administration Tip

Never recap used nonsafety syringes. Always discard the used syringes in appropriate disposal containers.

Reconstituting Powdered Medication

Sometimes the nurse has to reconstitute a powdered medication for intramuscular or intravenous administration. In such cases, always follow the label directions to achieve the correct dosage-to-solute ratio. See Figure 4-14.

M edication Administration Tip

When reconstituting a powdered medication, add the exact amount of diluting solution according to the label and then mix the solution by rolling the vial in the palms of the hands.

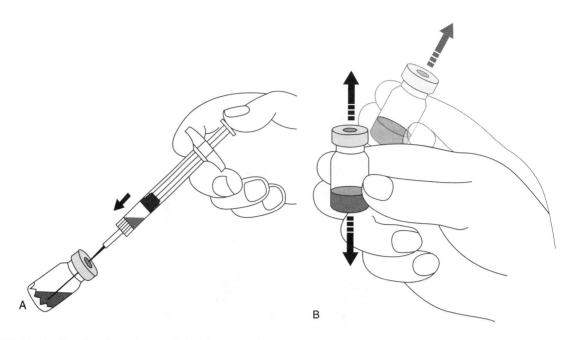

FIGURE 4-14   Powdered medication (A) before, and (B) after it has been reconstituted.

Adding Medications to Intravenous Solution Bags

Adding medications to intravenous solution bags must be done correctly and under sterile conditions. Review the following steps to learn how to safely add medications to intravenous solution bags:

1. Locate the injection port on the intravenous bag. Clean off the port using an antiseptic swab.

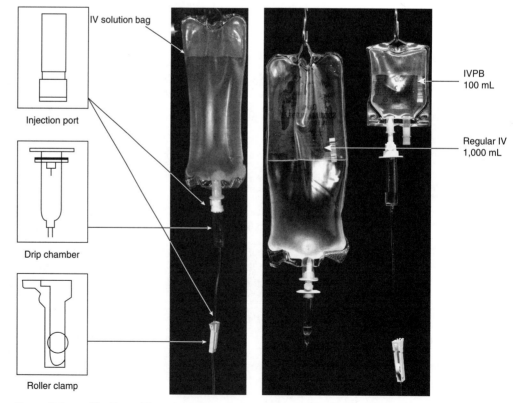

IV solution bag

Injection port

Drip chamber

Roller clamp

IVPB
100 mL

Regular IV
1,000 mL

Source: © George Allen Penton/ShutterStock, Inc.

Source: © Robert Byron/Dreamstime.com

2. Insert needle into the center of the injection port and inject medication. Remove needle and dispose of properly. Rotate the intravenous bag gently to mix medication and affix completed medication label.

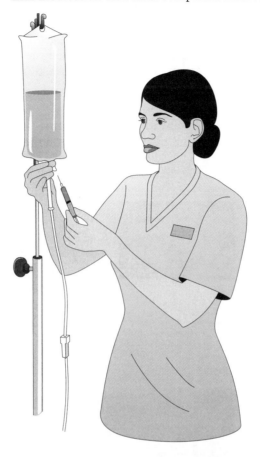

Drawing Up Two Types of Insulin in the Same Syringe

FIGURE 4-15 Roll the vial gently between the hands to warm the solution.

Insulin is a very fragile medication and can be easily destroyed with rough handling. So it is recommended that (see Figure 4-15):

- When you are warming cool insulin, gently roll the vial in the palms of the hands; do not shake it.
- When placing air into an insulin vial, inject the air into air, not into the solution.

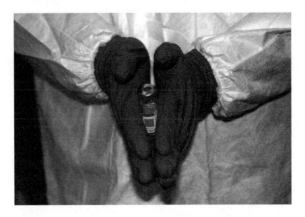

Also, when mixing two insulin solutions, follow these steps in the order shown:

1. Inject air into the air space in a vial of long-acting insulin.
2. Inject air into the air space of a vial of short-acting insulin.

3. Draw up the short-acting insulin.
4. Draw up the long-acting insulin.

The reason for this safety practice is to avoid harmful spillage of insulin from one vial to the other. If a minute amount of short-acting insulin happens to spill into the long-acting insulin, the action of the long-acting insulin remains relatively unchanged. Conversely, if a minute amount of long-acting insulin spills into the short-acting insulin, the action of the short-acting insulin could be dangerously altered.

POSTTEST

Remember to show all work and to proof all answers.
Questions 1–10: Circle the following on the medication labels.

1. Generic name of the drug

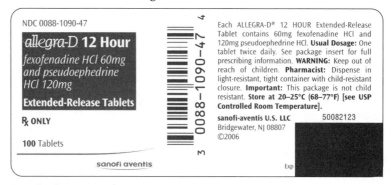

Source: © sanofi-aventis US. Used with permission.

2. Supply dosage

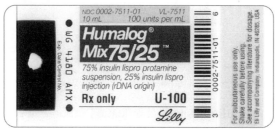

Source: © Eli Lilly and Company. Used with permission.

3. Expiration date

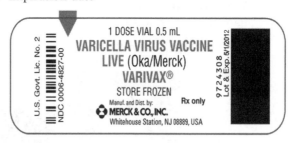

Source: Courtesy of Merck & Co., Inc.

4. Bar code

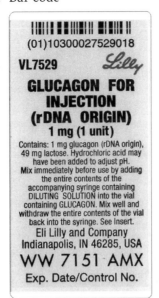

Source: © Eli Lilly and Company. Used with permission.

5. Storage instructions

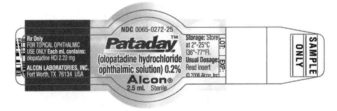

Source: © Alcon Laboratories, Inc. Used with permission.

6. Route of drug

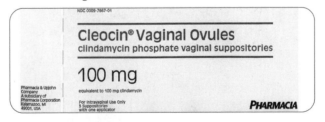

Source: © Pfizer Inc. Used with permission.

7. Number of dosages

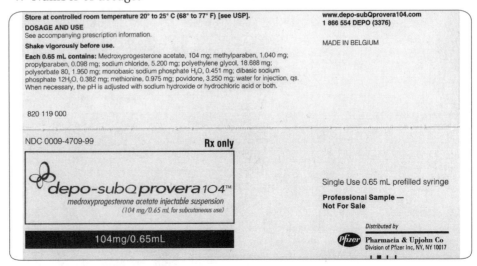

Source: © Pfizer Inc. Used with permission.

M edication Administration Tip

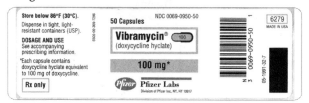

Depo-subQ Provera (medroxyprogesterone acetate) is a hormone/antineoplastic used in the treatment of reducing endometrial hyperplasia and long-acting contraception.

8. Drug form

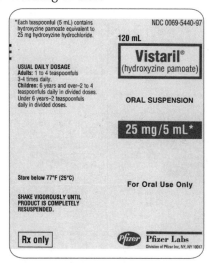

Source: © Pfizer Inc. Used with permission.

9. Warning or alert

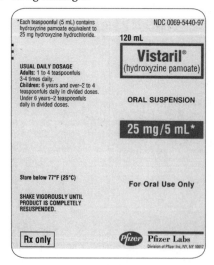

Source: © Pfizer Inc. Used with permission.

10. Drug strength

Source: © Pfizer Inc. Used with permission.

Questions 11–15: Shade the syringe with the correct dosage.

11. 18 units

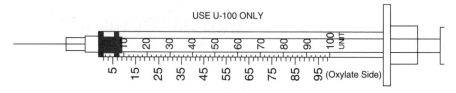

12. 10 minims

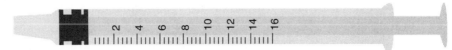

13. 1.8 milliliters

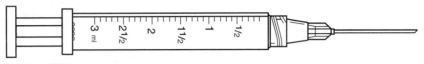

14. 3.25 milliliters.

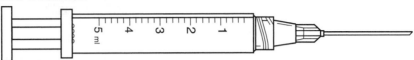

15. 6.7 milliliters

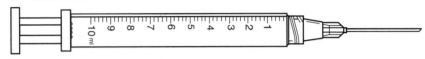

Questions 16–20: Answer the questions based on the clinical scenario provided.

Clinical Scenario

A client diagnosed with advanced cancer of the colon comes to the clinic with acute rectal bleeding with bowel movements. He is complaining of abdominal pain, he is afebrile, and slightly dehydrated. The clinic doctor orders 500 ml D5W with 1 ampule of multivitamin to infuse over the next 3 hours for rehydration, Eloxatin 100 mg IVPB as a one-time dose, and Demerol 50 mg IM Q4H PRN for pain.

---

*M*edication Administration Tip

> Eloxatin (oxaliplatin) is an antineoplastic agent used in the treatment of metastatic colon and rectal cancer.

16. What size syringe and needle would the healthcare provider select to administer the Demerol?
    a. 3 ml, 21 gauge, 1 inch
    b. 1 ml, 18 gauge, 1/2 inch
    c. 5 ml, 25 gauge, 5/8 inch
    d. 10 ml, 26 gauge, 1/2 inch

17. How many milliliters would the healthcare provider add to the Eloxatin vial to reconstitute the powered mixture?

    Answer: _____20_____ ml

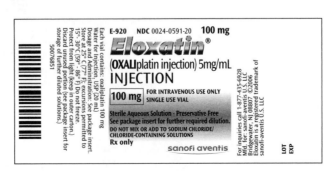

18. How many milliliters would the healthcare provider draw up to correctly administer the ordered amount of Eloxatin?

    Answer: ____20____ ml

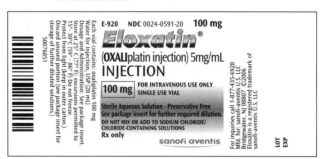

Source: © sanofi-aventis US. Used with permission.

19. How would the healthcare provider add the multivitamin to the empty intravenous bag of D5NS solution? Number the steps in the correct order.

    a. __c__ Rotate the bag.

    b. __d__ Inject the medication.

    c. __a__ Draw up the medication.

    d. __b__ Swab the IV bag port.

    e. __e__ Label the bag containing the multivitamin.

20. How would the healthcare provider draw up the client's morning insulin for administration? Ordered: 10 units of regular insulin and 15 units of NPH insulin. Number the steps in the correct order.

    a. __b__ Inject air into regular insulin.

    b. __a__ Inject air into NPH insulin.

    c. __d__ Draw up NPH insulin.

    d. __c__ Draw up regular insulin.

Answers

Answers to Practice Questions for Reading Medication Labels

1.

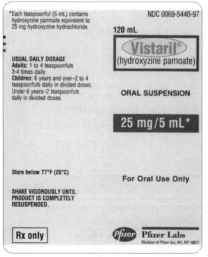

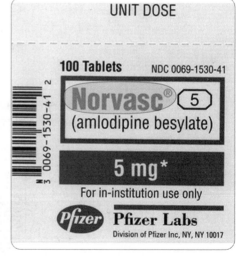

Source: © Pfizer Inc. Used with permission.

2.

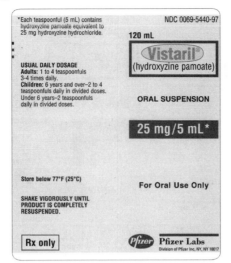

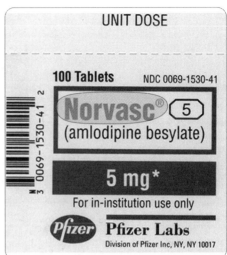

3.

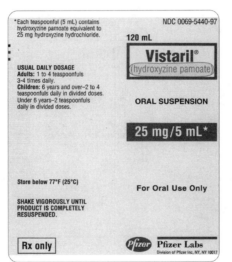

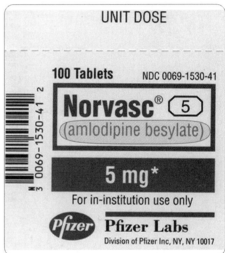

4.

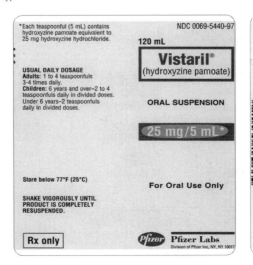

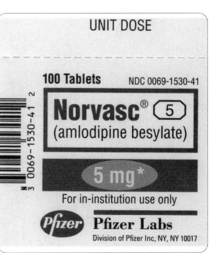

5.

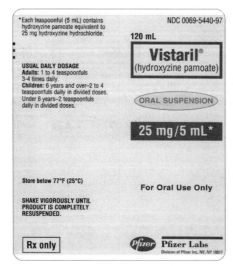

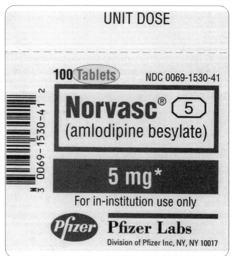

Source: © Pfizer Inc. Used with permission.

6.

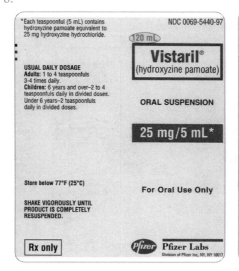

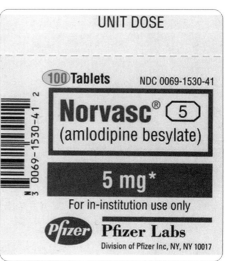

Source: © Pfizer Inc. Used with permission.

7.

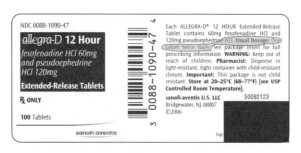

Source: © sanofi-aventis US. Used with permission.

Source: © sanofi-aventis US. Used with permission.

8.

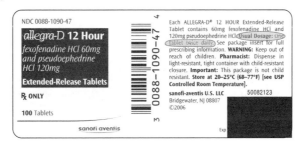

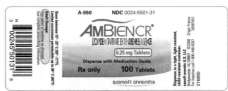

9.

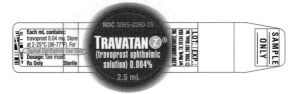

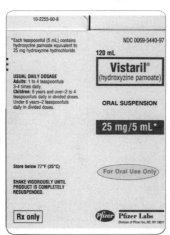

10.

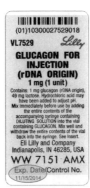

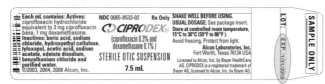

11.

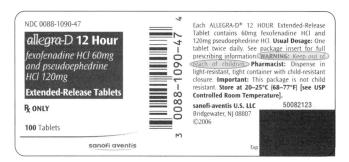

Source: © sanofi-aventis US. Used with permission.

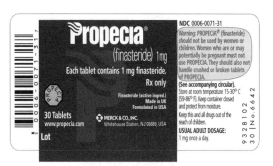

Source: Courtesy of Merck & Co., Inc.

12.

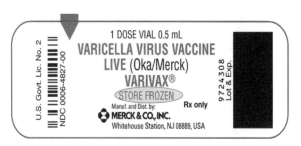

Source: Courtesy of Merck & Co., Inc.

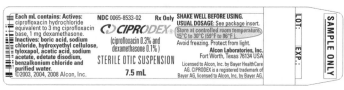

Source: © Alcon Laboratories, Inc. Used with permission.

13.

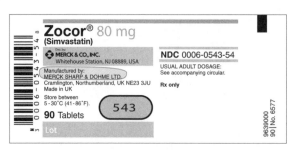

Source: Courtesy of Merck & Co., Inc.

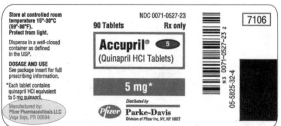

Source: © Pfizer Inc. Used with permission.

14.

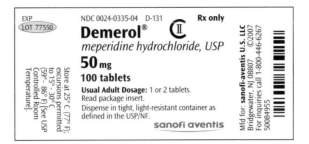

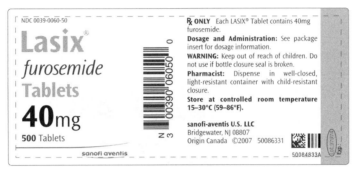

15.

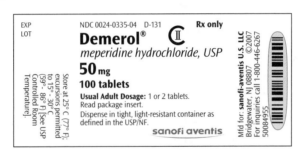

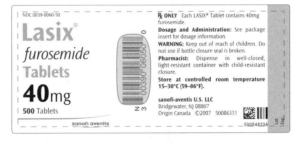

Answers to Practice Questions for Reading Injection Syringes

1. 17 units
2. 3 units
3. 10 units
4.

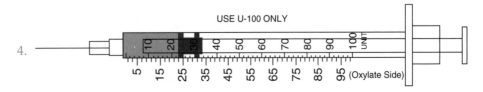

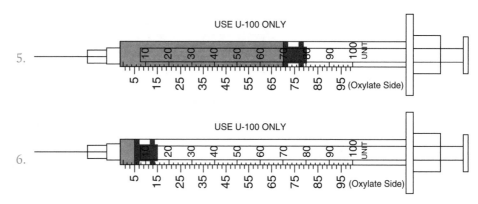

5.

6.

7. 16 minims

8. 8 minims

9. 3 minims

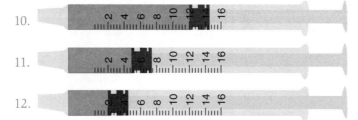

10.

11.

12.

13. 0.6 milliliters

14. 1.7 milliliters

15. 3.8 milliliters

16. 7.5 milliliters

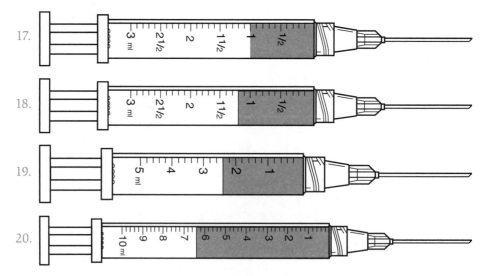

17.

18.

19.

20.

Answers to Posttest

1.

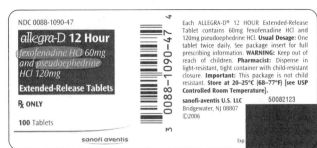

Source: © sanofi-aventis US. Used with permission.

2.

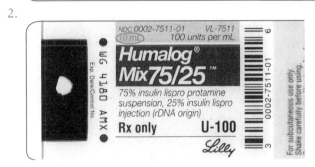

Source: © Eli Lilly and Company. Used with permission.

3.

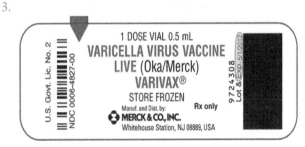

Source: Courtesy of Merck & Co., Inc.

4.

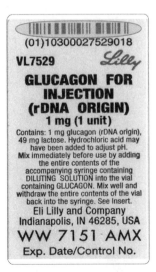

Source: © Eli Lilly and Company. Used with permission.

5.

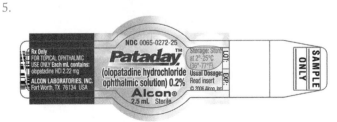

Source: © Alcon Laboratories, Inc. Used with permission.

6.

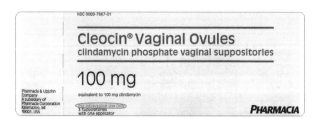

7.

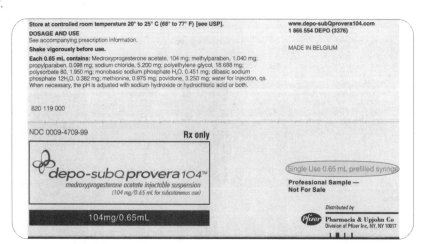

8.

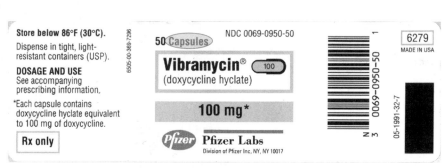

9.

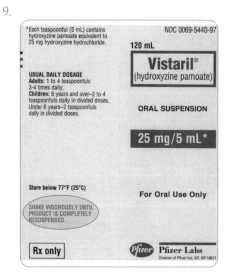

10.

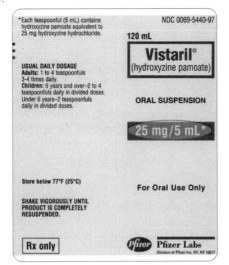

Source: © Pfizer Inc. Used with
permission.

11.

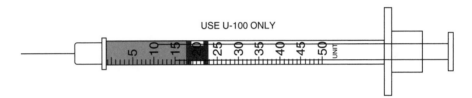

12.

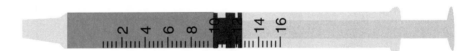

13.

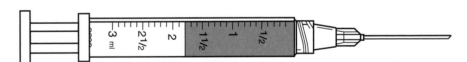

14.

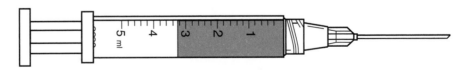

15.

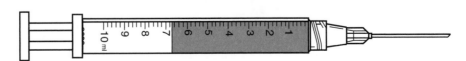

16. a
17. 20 ml
18. 20 ml
19. c, d, a, b, and e.
20. b, a, d, and c.

Reference

Potter, A. P., & Perry, A. G. (2005). *Fundamentals of nursing.* Philadelphia: Mosby.

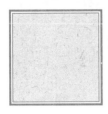

5 Executing Physician's Orders

Introduction

This chapter is designed to assist you in

- Reading the physician's order correctly
- Reading prescription orders correctly
- Questioning drug orders
- Identifying various types of physician orders
  - Routine
  - PRN
  - Single dose
  - STAT
- Practicing the skill of interpreting physician's written medication orders
- Completing a chapter posttest

Reading the Physician's Order

Reading a physician's order accurately is a vital part of giving medications safely. The physician's order must be stamped or labeled with the client's name, contain complete information as to drug, dose, route, and time, and be legible. Nurses and allied health professionals practice the art of reading doctors' orders, which can sometimes be stressful. A correct physician's order has multiple parts. See Figure 5-1.

When reading a doctor's order, you should ask yourself questions like the following:

- Are the client's name, the date, and allergy fields filled in?
- Is the name of the medication written clearly?
- Are dosage, drug form, route, and times listed?

If any of this information is missing, contact the ordering physician to get it. To administer any medication without complete information is malpractice.

Practice Question on Reading the Order

In Figure 5-2, circle the following information:

- Date
- Client name

FIGURE 5-1   Doctor's order sheet.

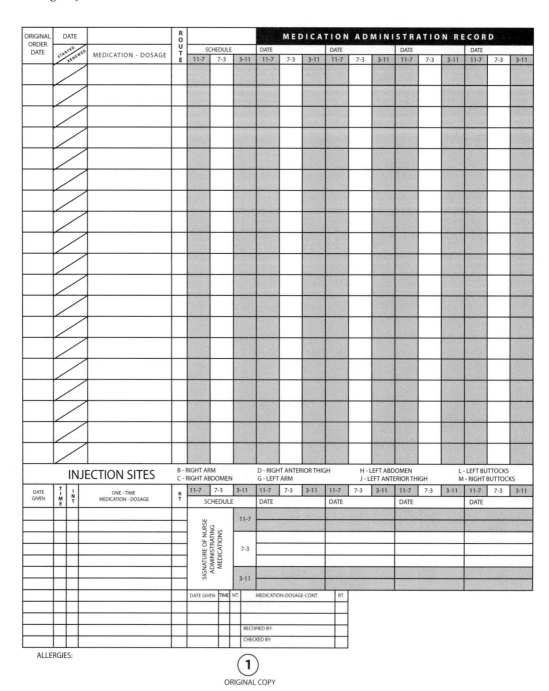

- Client allergies
- Medication names
- Medication dosages
- Drug form
- Drug route
- Time and frequency of administration

FIGURE 5-2 Completed doctor's order sheet.

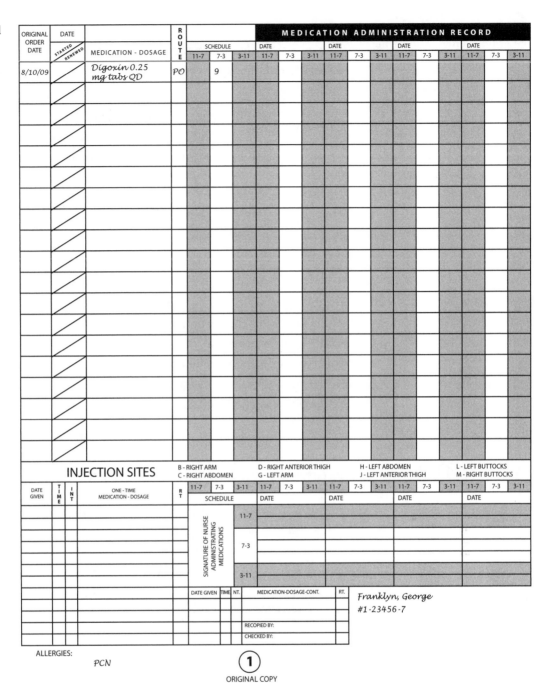

Physician's Prescription Orders

Physicians often require clients to take medications at home and will complete a prescription order form for the client to give to the pharmacist. A correctly filled-out prescription form should include (see Figure 5-3):

• The superscription, which includes the client's name, age, address, birthday, and contact number.

• The Rx, meaning "to take."

FIGURE 5-3 A completed prescription order includes the client's name, date of birth, sex, and date of ordering. It also includes the inscription (the medication and dosage), the subscription (what is to be dispensed), and the sigma sig (how the medication is to be taken). The number of refills should be filled out and directions to "dispense as written" (DAW) if generic medications are unacceptable. The ordering healthcare provider must sign the prescription.

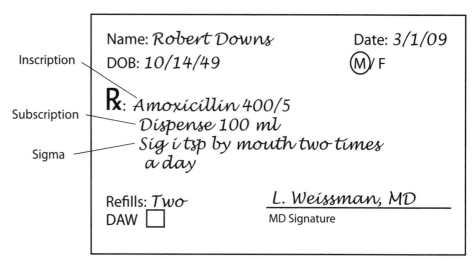

* The signature, which includes the drug name, strength, dosage to take, and any directions the client needs.
* The number of refills.
* Other information, including whether an easy-open top is needed.
* The order to dispense as written.
* The physician's signature.

Types of Orders

Nurses and allied health care professionals deal directly with various types of orders:

* *Routine medication orders* (also known as *standing orders*) are carried out until the ordering healthcare provider discontinues the medication.

■ **EXAMPLE:**

Mecamylamine hydrochloride (Inversine) 2.5 mg BID. This medication is given every day, twice a day. ■

M edication Administration Tip

Mecamylamine hydrochloride (Inversine) is an antihypertensive used to treat moderately severe to severe hypertension and malignant hypertension.

* *PRN orders* (also known as *as-needed orders*) are carried out as the client needs the medication. As an example, medication ordered for pain is administered as ordered when the client requests it or as the healthcare provider assesses it is necessary.

■ EXAMPLE: Oxycodone hydrochloride and ibuprofen 5 mg/ 400 mg PO Q6H PRN as needed for pain. This medication is administered every 6 hours if the client has pain. In the absence of pain, the medication is not given. ▪

M edication Administration Tip

> Oxycodone hydrochloride and ibuprofen (Combunox) is an analgesic combination drug used to treat short-term acute, moderate to severe pain.

- *Single-dose orders* (also known as *one-time orders*) are for a single administration and then the order is cancelled.

■ EXAMPLE: Atropine 0.4 mg intramuscularly on call to the operating room × one dose. This medication is given when the client is taken to the surgical unit. ▪

M edication Administration Tip

> Atropine (AtroPen) is an anticholinergic, antimuscarinic used to reduce respiratory tract secretions related to anesthesia.

- *STAT orders* (also known as *immediate orders*) are administered without delay. Very often the medications are of a lifesaving nature.

■ EXAMPLE: Lidocaine hydrochloride 50 mg intravenous push STAT × one dose. This medication is administered immediately. ▪

M edication Administration Tip

> Lidocaine hydrochloride is a Class IB antiarrhythmic used to treat ventricular tachycardia or ventricular fibrillation.

Posttest   Practice Questions for Physician's Medication Orders

Read the following medication orders and answer the questions.

Sample Drug Order 1

ORIGINAL ORDER DATE	DATE STARTED/RENEWED	MEDICATION - DOSAGE	ROUTE	SCHEDULE 11-7	7-3	3-11	MEDICATION ADMINISTRATION RECORD DATE 11-7	7-3	3-11	DATE 11-7	7-3	3-11	DATE 11-7	7-3	3-11	DATE 11-7	7-3	3-11
1/3/09		Keflex 500 mg tabs QID	PO		9A	5P												
					1P	9P												

INJECTION SITES

B - RIGHT ARM C - RIGHT ABDOMEN D - RIGHT ANTERIOR THIGH G - LEFT ARM H - LEFT ABDOMEN J - LEFT ANTERIOR THIGH L - LEFT BUTTOCKS M - RIGHT BUTTOCKS

DATE GIVEN	TIME	INT	ONE - TIME MEDICATION - DOSAGE	RT	11-7	7-3	3-11	11-7	7-3	3-11	11-7	7-3	3-11	11-7	7-3	3-11	11-7	7-3	3-11
					SCHEDULE			DATE			DATE			DATE			DATE		

SIGNATURE OF NURSE ADMINISTERING MEDICATIONS

	11-7
	7-3
	3-11

DATE GIVEN	TIME	NT.	MEDICATION-DOSAGE-CONT.	RT.

Cole, Alice
#2-34567-8

RECOPIED BY:

CHECKED BY:

ALLERGIES:
NKDA

(1)
ORIGINAL COPY

1. What is the client's name? _____
2. Does the client have any allergies? _____
3. What is the date of the order? _____
4. What is the name of the medication ordered? _____
5. What is the dose of the drug? _____

6. What is the form of the drug? _____

7. What is the route of the drug? _____

8. What time should you administer the drug? _____

Sample Drug Order 2

ORIGINAL ORDER DATE	DATE STARTED / RENEWED	MEDICATION - DOSAGE	R O U T E	SCHEDULE			MEDICATION ADMINISTRATION RECORD											
							DATE			DATE			DATE			DATE		
				11-7	7-3	3-11	11-7	7-3	3-11	11-7	7-3	3-11	11-7	7-3	3-11	11-7	7-3	3-11
3/10/09		Atenolol 100mg caps qam	po		9A													

INJECTION SITES
B - RIGHT ARM   D - RIGHT ANTERIOR THIGH   H - LEFT ABDOMEN   L - LEFT BUTTOCKS
C - RIGHT ABDOMEN   G - LEFT ARM   J - LEFT ANTERIOR THIGH   M - RIGHT BUTTOCKS

DATE GIVEN	TIME	INT	ONE - TIME MEDICATION - DOSAGE	RT	11-7	7-3	3-11	11-7	7-3	3-11	qam 11-7	7-3	3-11	11-7	7-3	3-11	11-7	7-3	3-11
					SCHEDULE			DATE			DATE			DATE			DATE		

SIGNATURE OF NURSE ADMINISTRATING MEDICATIONS: 11-7 / 7-3 / 3-11

DATE GIVEN	TIME	NT.	MEDICATION-DOSAGE-CONT.	RT.

Donnell, Robert
#3-45678-9

RECOPIED BY:
CHECKED BY:

ALLERGIES: *ASA*

(**1**)
ORIGINAL COPY

9. What is the client's name? _____

10. Does the client have any allergies? _____

11. What is the date of the order? _____

12. What is the name of the medication ordered? _____

13. What is the dose of the drug? _____

14. What is the form of the drug? _____

15. What is the route of the drug? _____

16. What time should you administer the drug? _____

Sample Drug Order 3

ORIGINAL ORDER DATE	DATE STARTED / RENEWED	MEDICATION - DOSAGE	R O U T E	SCHEDULE 11-7 / 7-3 / 3-11	MEDICATION ADMINISTRATION RECORD
4/5/09		Regular insulin 20u qam AC	SQ	7A	

INJECTION SITES

B - RIGHT ARM	D - RIGHT ANTERIOR THIGH	H - LEFT ABDOMEN	L - LEFT BUTTOCKS
C - RIGHT ABDOMEN	G - LEFT ARM	J - LEFT ANTERIOR THIGH	M - RIGHT BUTTOCKS

DATE GIVEN	TIME	INT	ONE - TIME MEDICATION - DOSAGE	RT	11-7 / 7-3 / 3-11 SCHEDULE			

SIGNATURE OF NURSE ADMINISTRATING MEDICATIONS 11-7 / 7-3 / 3-11

DATE GIVEN	TIME	NT.	MEDICATION-DOSAGE-CONT.	RT.

Johns, Margaret
#4-56789-0

RECOPIED BY:
CHECKED BY:

ALLERGIES:

Shrimp, crab

(1)
ORIGINAL COPY

17. What is the client's name? _____

18. Does the client have any allergies? _____

19. What is the date of the order? _____

20. What is the name of the medication ordered? _____

21. What is the dose of the drug? _____

22. What is the form of the drug? _____

23. What is the route of the drug? _____
24. What time should you administer the drug? _____

Sample Drug Order 4

ORIGINAL ORDER DATE	DATE STARTED / RENEWED	MEDICATION - DOSAGE	ROUTE	SCHEDULE			MEDICATION ADMINISTRATION RECORD											
							DATE			DATE			DATE			DATE		
				11-7	7-3	3-11	11-7	7-3	3-11	11-7	7-3	3-11	11-7	7-3	3-11	11-7	7-3	3-11
5/5/09		Gentamycin 1 gm q6h	IV PB	12MN 6A	12N	6P												

INJECTION SITES

B - RIGHT ARM   D - RIGHT ANTERIOR THIGH   H - LEFT ABDOMEN   L - LEFT BUTTOCKS
C - RIGHT ABDOMEN   G - LEFT ARM   J - LEFT ANTERIOR THIGH   M - RIGHT BUTTOCKS

DATE GIVEN	TIME	INT	ONE - TIME MEDICATION - DOSAGE	RT	11-7	7-3	3-11	11-7	7-3	3-11	11-7	7-3	3-11	11-7	7-3	3-11
					SCHEDULE			DATE			DATE			DATE		

SIGNATURE OF NURSE ADMINISTRATING MEDICATIONS

	11-7
	7-3
	3-11

DATE GIVEN	TIME	NT.	MEDICATION-DOSAGE-CONT.	RT.

Marzilla, Lori
#0-12345-6

RECOPIED BY:
CHECKED BY:

ALLERGIES: Latex

(1)
ORIGINAL COPY

25. What is the client's name? _____
26. Does the client have any allergies? _____
27. What is the date of the order? _____
28. What is the name of the medication ordered? _____
29. What is the dose of the drug? _____
30. What is the form of the drug? _____

31. What is the route of the drug? _____

32. What time should you administer the drug? _____

Sample Drug Order 5

ORIGINAL ORDER DATE	DATE STARTED/RENEWED	MEDICATION - DOSAGE	ROUTE	SCHEDULE 11-7	7-3	3-11	DATE 11-7	7-3	3-11	DATE 11-7	7-3	3-11	DATE 11-7	7-3	3-11	DATE 11-7	7-3	3-11
		MEDICATION ADMINISTRATION RECORD																
6/1/09		Timoptin eye drops 2gtts BID	OU		9A	5P												

INJECTION SITES

B - RIGHT ARM	D - RIGHT ANTERIOR THIGH	H - LEFT ABDOMEN	L - LEFT BUTTOCKS	
C - RIGHT ABDOMEN	G - LEFT ARM	J - LEFT ANTERIOR THIGH	M - RIGHT BUTTOCKS	

DATE GIVEN	TIME	INT	ONE - TIME MEDICATION - DOSAGE	RT	11-7	7-3	3-11	11-7	7-3	3-11	11-7	7-3	3-11	11-7	7-3	3-11	11-7	7-3	3-11
					SCHEDULE			DATE			DATE			DATE			DATE		

SIGNATURE OF NURSE ADMINISTRATING MEDICATIONS

11-7

7-3

3-11

DATE GIVEN	TIME	NT.	MEDICATION-DOSAGE-CONT.	RT.

Webster, Rebecca
#9-87654-3

RECOPIED BY:

CHECKED BY:

ALLERGIES:

NKA

(1)
ORIGINAL COPY

33. What is the client's name? _____

34. Does the client have any allergies? _____

35. What is the date of the order? _____

36. What is the name of the medication ordered? _____

37. What is the dose of the drug? _____

38. What is the form of the drug? _____

39. What is the route of the drug? _____

40. What time should you administer the drug? _____

Practice Questions for Questioning Medication Orders

Read the following physician's orders, select the medication order you would question, and state why you would question it.

41. The doctor orders iron supplements for your client, who is diagnosed with anemia, to be given every morning with a glass of milk. What in this order would you question and why?

_____   _____

_____   _____

_____   _____

42. The physician orders Tylenol 2 tablets PO for the client preoperatively. The client has been prepped and has been NPO since midnight. What in this order would you question and why?

_____   _____

_____   _____

_____   _____

43. A client is scheduled for an intravenous pyelogram (IVP). He has been fasting since the night before and is nervous. He tells you he is allergic to penicillin and shrimp. The physician orders an IV of D5W to run at a keep-vein-open (KVO) rate and an injection of IVP dye on call to the x-ray department. What in this order would you question and why?

_____   _____

_____   _____

_____   _____

44. A client comes to the clinic to have a colonoscopy with possible biopsy. The client states that she has not eaten anything this morning and that she took her medications with a few sips of water, as instructed by her doctor. When reviewing exactly what medications she took, you discover she has taken her digoxin, Lasix, and Coumadin. What in this order would you question and why?

_____   _____

_____   _____

_____   _____

45. A doctor orders Demerol 500 mg intramuscularly for a postoperative male client. The client tells the nurse his pain scale is 9 out of 10. He is NPO, and his vital

signs are stable. He has not had pain medication since returning from the post-anesthesia care unit (PACU). What in this order would you question and why?

_____   _____

_____   _____

_____   _____

Answers

Answers to Posttest Practice Questions for Physician's Orders

Sample Drug Order 1

1. Alice Cole
2. No known drug allergies
3. 1/3/09
4. Keflex

5. 500 mg
6. Tablets
7. PO
8. 9 am, 1 pm, 5 pm, 9 pm

Sample Drug Order 2

9. Robert Donnell
10. ASA (aspirin)
11. 3/10/09
12. Atenolol

13. 100 mg
14. Capsules
15. PO
16. 9 am

Sample Drug Order 3

17. Margaret Johns
18. Shrimp, crab
19. 4/5/09
20. Regular insulin

21. 20 u
22. Injectable
23. Subcutaneous
24. 7 am before breakfast

Sample Drug Order 4

25. Lori Marzilla
26. Latex
27. 5/5/09
28. Gentamycin

29. 1 gm
30. Intravenous
31. Intravenous piggy-back
32. 12 midnight, 6 am, 12 noon, 6 pm

Sample Drug Order 5

33. Rebecca Webster
34. No known allergies
35. 6/1/09
36. Timoptin eye drops

37. 2 gtts each eye
38. Liquid eye drops
39. Eye medication (each eye)
40. 9 am, 5 pm

Answers to Practice Questions for Questioning Medication Orders

41. Iron preparations are usually given with fluids high in vitamin C, such as orange juice, not milk. The iron binds with the vitamin C, increasing absorption.

42. The client is NPO (nothing by mouth) and should not be given Tylenol 2 orally.

43. The client is allergic to shrimp, and the IVP dye has an iodine base. The risk of an allergic reaction is increased in clients with seafood allergies.

44. A colonoscopy with biopsy may cause bleeding, and the client should not take Coumadin and other blood thinners for 1 week prior to the procedure. The risk of hemorrhage is increased.

45. Demerol 500 mg is considered a lethal dose. The usual dose is 25 mg up to 100 mg intramuscularly for pain.

6 Intravenous Solutions and Medication Administration

Introduction

The preparation and administration of intravenous solutions are integral to medication administration for all healthcare professionals. There are various types of intravenous solutions in a number of sizes. A host of medications can be added to fluids. See Figure 6-1.

This chapter is designed to assist you in calculating:

- Intravenous dosages
- Milliliters per hour
- Drops per minute
- Total time (TT) in minutes

This chapter will also assist you in:

- Identifying types and sizes of various intravenous solution bags
- Spiking an IV bag
- Identifying intravenous tubing sets

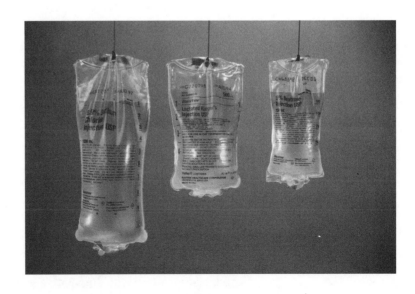

FIGURE 6-1 Intravenous solutions come in different types and sizes.

M *edication Administration Tip*

Spiking an intravenous solution bag, a sterile procedure, can be accomplished by carefully following these steps (Potter & Perry, 2005, pp. 1182–1183):

* Perform hand hygiene.
* Move the roller clamp to the closed position on the tubing.
* Remove the cover from the tubing spike.
* Insert the spike into the solution bag.
* Hang the bag on the IV pole.
* Squeeze the chamber to fill it one-third to one-half with solution.
* Open the clamp and prime the tubing, being careful to fill the tubing slowly and to avoid air bubbles.
* Proceed to administer the solution.

See Figure 6-2.

FIGURE 6-2 IV bag with port and IV tubing.

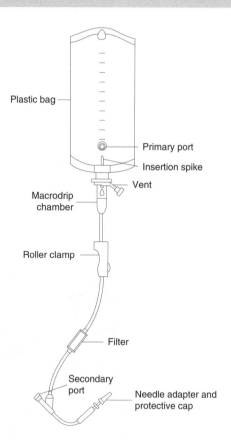

Plastic bag

Primary port

Insertion spike

Vent

Macrodrip chamber

Roller clamp

Filter

Secondary port

Needle adapter and protective cap

M *edication Administration Tip*

The correct selection and preparation of IV equipment assist in the safe and quick placement of an IV line (Potter & Perry, 2005, p. 1161).

Calculating Intravenous Dosages

You must take two main steps when calculating intravenous fluids for administration.

1. Calculate the amount of fluid to be administered.
2. Calculate the dosage of the medication to be given in the fluid intravenously.

Specifically, the steps to follow are to:

1. Determine how many milliliters per hour to infuse.
2. Calculate the drops per minute.

Step 1: Milliliters per Hour

To calculate the ml per hour, use the following formula:

$$\frac{\text{Total volume}}{\text{Total time (in hours)}} = \text{Infusion rate per hour (ml/hr)}$$

■ **EXAMPLE:**

The doctor has ordered the client to receive 2000 ml of D5W intravenously in the next 24 hours. See Table 6-1.

$$\frac{\text{Total volume (TV)}}{\text{Total time (TT, in hours)}} = \text{Infusion rate per hour}$$

$$\frac{2000\ \text{ml}}{24\ \text{hr}} = 83\ \text{ml/hr for 24 hr}$$

The client needs to have 83 milliliters of fluid infused every hour for the next 24 hours. ■

TABLE 6-1   **Acceptable Abbreviations for Frequently Used Intravenous Solutions**

RL	**Ringer's lactate**
NS	Normal saline 0.9%
$^1/_2$ NS	Normal saline 0.45%
$^1/_4$ NS	Normal saline 0.225%
D5W and 5%DW	Dextrose 5% in water
D5NS	Dextrose 5% in normal saline
D5RL	Dextrose 5% in Ringer's lactate
D10W and 10%DW	Dextrose 10% in water

Step 2: Drops per Minute

Now that you know how many milliliters the client needs to have per hour, you need to calculate the drops per minute (gtts).

The Drop Factor

First determine the drop factor of the intravenous tubing you are using. The package the tubing comes in should have the drop factor written in bold letters or numbers. Sometimes the drop factor is written on the outside of the chamber or on one of the tubing clamps. The drop factor determines how many drops it takes to deliver 1 milliliter of solution.

■ **EXAMPLE:**

A drop factor of 10 indicates that when 10 drops are delivered, the client has received 1 ml of fluid. A drop factor of 15 indicates the client will receive 1 ml of fluid when 15 drops have been delivered. There are also tubing sets with drop factors of 20 and 60. ■

Tubing with a drop factor of 60 is referred to as microtubing due to the fact that the drops are very small. When calculating the drops per minute for microtubing, remember that the milliliters per hour and the drops per minute are the same. For example, an intravenous running at 100 milliliters per hour with a microtubing administration set would be set at 100 drops per minute.

The Drops per Minute Formulas

When the time is in *hours*, the formula for calculating drops per minute is

$$\frac{\text{Total volume (TV)}}{\text{Total time (TT, in hours)}} \times \frac{\text{Drop factor}}{60 \text{ minutes}} = \text{Drops per minute}$$

The drop factor is over 60 when the total time is in hours, indicating that the time is to be changed into minutes (60 minutes = 1 hour). Remember, the answer to the formula is in gtts per minute.

When the time is in *minutes*, the formula for calculating drops per minute is

$$\frac{\text{Total volume (TV)}}{\text{Total time (TT, in minutes)}} \times \frac{\text{Drop factor}}{1} = \text{Drops per minute}$$

The drop factor is over 1 when the total time is already in minutes and no time conversion is necessary.

■ **EXAMPLE:**

Now that you know the client needs to have 83 milliliters of fluid, you need to calculate the drops per minute. The general formula is

$$\frac{\text{Total volume (TV)}}{\text{Total time (TT, in hours)}} \times \frac{\text{Drop factor}}{60 \text{ minutes}} = \text{Drops per minute}$$

If you are using microtubing (a drop factor of 60), then:

$$\frac{83 \text{ ml/hr}}{1 \text{ hr}} \times \frac{60}{60 \text{ min}} = 83 \text{ gtts per minute}$$

Here's another example:

■ **EXAMPLE:**

The doctor's orders are for 500 ml D5W to infuse in 5 hours. Microtubing is used.

Step 1:

$$\frac{500 \text{ ml}}{5 \text{ hr}} 5 = 100 \text{ ml/hr}$$

Step 2:

$$\frac{100 \text{ ml}}{60 \text{ min}} \times \frac{60}{1} = 100 \text{ gtts/min}$$

M edication Administration Tip

Intravenous pumps or volume control devices are crucial when administering medications that require precise rates. Such devices are recommended to use with all clients receiving intravenous fluids to prevent fluid overload and/or medication overdosing. See Figure 6-3.

FIGURE 6-3 Standard infusion set with volume control chamber.

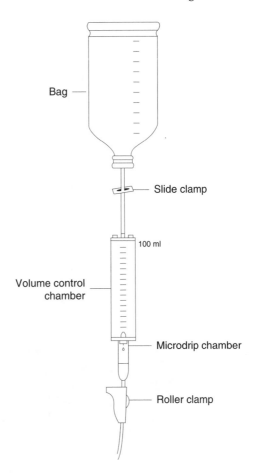

Bag

Slide clamp

100 ml

Volume control chamber

Microdrip chamber

Roller clamp

Practice Questions for Calculating Milliliters per Hour

The formula for calculating the infusion rate (milliliters per hour) is

$$\frac{\text{Total volume (TV)}}{\text{Total time (TT, in hours)}} = \text{Infusion rate per hour (ml/hr)}$$

Using this formula, solve the following problems. Remember to show all work and to proof all answers.

1. A client is to receive 100 milliliters of dextrose 10% water intravenously over a 20-minute period. At what rate should the IV pump be set? (Most IV pumps are set in milliliters per hour.)

2. A client is to receive 500 milliliters Ringer's lactate intravenously every 8 hours. At what rate should the nurse administer the solution?

3. The doctor orders 1000 milliliters of dextrose 5% water, 1000 milliliters dextrose and normal saline, and 1000 milliliters Ringer's lactate intravenously to run in 24 hours. For how many milliliters per hour should the healthcare worker set the pump?

4. A client's intravenous of dextrose and 0.225% normal saline has 650 milliliters left to run. The MD orders the nurse to infuse the remaining fluid over the next 3 hours and then discontinue the IV. How many milliliters per hour should the nurse infuse for the following 3 hours?

5. You have an order to infuse 1000 milliliters of dextrose 5% water beginning at 9 am and ending at 2 pm. At what rate will you set the IV pump?

Practice Questions for Calculating Drops per Minute

The two formulas for calculating drops per minute are

$$\frac{\text{Total volume (TV)}}{\text{Total time (TT, in hours)}} \times \frac{\text{Drop factor}}{60 \text{ minutes}} = \text{Drops per minute}$$

$$\frac{\text{Total volume (TV)}}{\text{Total time (TT, in minutes)}} \times \frac{\text{Drop factor}}{1} = \text{Drops per minute}$$

With these formulas in mind, calculate drops per minute in the following problems. Remember to show all work and to proof all answers.

1. The doctor orders 1000 ml dextrose 5% normal saline to infuse in 8 hr. The drop factor on the tubing is 10 gtts/ml. You will give

    _____ml/hr   _____gtts/min

R *ounding Answers*

General practice is to round answers for medication administration when calculating intravenous solutions. If the answer is 0.5 or more (such as 20.6), round up to the nearest whole number (21). If the answer is 0.4 or less (such as 20.2), round down to the lowest whole number (20).

2. The doctor orders 100 ml intravenous piggyback (IVPB) to run in 15 minutes. The drop factor on the tubing is 20 gtts/ml. You will give

    _____gtts/min

3. The surgeon orders 1500 Ringer's lactate intravenously for a postoperative client to infuse in 10 hours. The drop factor on the tubing is 15 gtts/ml. You will give

    _____ml/hr   _____gtts/min

4. The nurse–midwife orders 2 liters of normal saline to infuse in 12 hours. The nurse uses microtubing. You will give

    _____ml/hr   _____gtts/min

5. The MD orders 75 ml of 0.9% normal saline to infuse in 30 min. The drop factor on the tubing is 20 gtts/ml. You will give

    _____gtts/min

Calculating Intravenous Solutions with Medication Added

When adding medication to an intravenous bag, the healthcare provider is responsible for determining the amount of fluid to be infused to deliver the ordered amount of the drug. For example, a physician orders 100 mg of a medication to be added to 1000 ml of IV fluid and administered at a rate of 10 mg per hour. The healthcare provider must first determine how many milliliters of fluid contain 10 mg of medication, which translates into the ml per hour to deliver, and second must determine the drops per minute.

Practice Questions for Calculating Intravenous Infusions with Added Medication

Solve the following problems. Remember to show all work and to proof all answers.

1. The doctor orders 500 ml of D5W with 100 units of regular insulin added to run at a rate of 10 units per hour. The drop factor on the tubing is 60 gtts/ml. You will give

   _____ ml/hr   _____ gtts/min

> Did you remember that when using microtubing the milliliters per hour and gtts per minute are the same?

2. The doctor orders 1000 ml of D5NS with 1,000,000 units of Pen VK to run at a rate of 100,000 units per hour. The drop factor on the tubing is 20 gtts/ml. You will give

   _____ ml/hr   _____ gtts/min

M edication Administration Tip

> Intravenous line maintenance is achieved by the following measures (Potter & Perry, 2005, p. 1180):
>
> * Keep the system sterile.
> * Change solutions, tubings, and site dressings according to agency protocol.
> * Assist the client with activities that might disrupt the system.

POSTTEST

Remember to show all work and to proof all answers.

1. *Ordered:* 250 ml DRL to be infused in 90 min

   Drop factor: microtubing

   Give: _____ gtts/min

2. *Ordered:* 1000 ml NS to be infused in 8 hr

   Drop factor: 10

   Give: _____ gtts/min

3. *Ordered:* 250 ml DRL to be infused in 1 hr

   Drop factor: 15

   Give: _____ gtts/min

4. *Ordered:* 50 ml NS to be infused in 20 min

   Drop factor: 60

   Give: _____ gtts/min

5. *Ordered:* 1500 ml D5W to be infused in 12 hr
   Drop factor: 20
   Give: _____ gtts/min

6. *Ordered:* 3000 ml D5%$^1/_2$NS to be infused in 24 hr
   Give: _____ ml/hr

7. *Ordered:* 1500 ml D5%$^1/_4$NS to be infused in 8 hr
   Give: _____ ml/hr

8. *Ordered:* 500 ml D5RL to be infused in 1 hr
   Give: _____ ml/hr

9. *Ordered:* 75 ml 0.9NS to be infused in 30 min
   Give: _____ ml/hr

10. *Ordered:* 1000 ml 0.225NS to be infused in 6 hr
    Give: _____ ml/hr

11. *Ordered:* 750 ml D5RL to be infused in 8 hr
    Drop factor: 60
    Give: _____ ml/hr   _____ gtts/min

12. *Ordered:* 2500 ml D5NS to be infused in 15 hr
    Drop factor: 15
    Give: _____ ml/hr   _____ gtts/min

13. Ordered 3000 ml D5W to be infused in 24 hr
    Drop factor: 10
    Give: _____ ml/hr   _____ gtts/min

14. *Ordered:* 500 ml 0.45NS to be infused in 12 hr
    Drop factor: 20
    Give: _____ ml/hr   _____ gtts/min

15. *Ordered:* 1 g Kefzol in 100 ml D5W to be infused in 30 min
    Drop factor: 60
    Give: _____ ml/hr   _____ gtts/min

16. *Ordered:* 1000 ml RL to be infused at 100 ml/hr
    Drop factor: 10
    Give: _____ ml/hr   _____ gtts/min

17. 1000 ml D^1/$_4$NS to be infused at 75 ml/hr

    Drop factor: 15

    Give: _____ ml/hr   _____ gtts/min

18. *Ordered:* 250 ml ^{1}/$_4$NS to be infused in 2 hr

    Drop factor: microtubing

    Give: _____ ml/hr   _____ gtts/min

19. *Ordered:* 500 ml DRL to be infused in 12 hr

    Drop factor: 15

    Give: _____ ml/hr   _____ gtts/min

20. *Ordered:* 800 ml NS left in the bottle (LIB) to be infused in 4 hr

    Drop factor: microtubing

    Give: _____ ml/hr   _____ gtts/min

21. *Ordered:* 1000 ml RL with 40 mEq KCl to be infused at a rate of 4 mEq/hr

    Drop factor: 15

    Give: _____ ml/hr   _____ gtts/min

22. *Ordered:* 400 ml D5^1/$_2$NS with 1 gram of an antibiotic to run at a rate of 100 mg of antibiotic per hour

    Drop factor: 15

    Give: _____ ml/hr   _____ gtts/min

23. *Ordered:* 100 ml NS with 500 mg Kefzol to infuse at a rate of 500 mg/hr

    Drop factor: microtubing

    Give: _____ ml/hr   _____ gtts/min

24. *Ordered:* 500 ml D5RL with 1 grain of a medication to infuse at 3 mg/hr

    Drop factor: 60

    Give: _____ ml/hr   _____ gtts/min

25. *Ordered:* 1000 ml of D5^1/$_4$NS with 1 gram of gentamicin to infuse at a rate of 150 mg/hr

    Drop factor: 10

    Give: _____ ml/hr   _____ gtts/min

M edication Administration Tip

An infiltration occurs when IV fluids enter space surrounding the venipuncture site. An indication of an infiltration includes (Potter & Perry, 2005, p. 1189):

- Swelling
- Pallor
- Coolness

Answers

Answers to Practice Questions for Calculating Milliliters per Hour

1. *Answer:* 300 milliliters per hour

   Solution: 100 ml ÷ 20 min = 100 ml ÷ 0.3 hr = 300 ml/hr

   Rationale: The 20 minutes must be converted to hours, and 20 minutes are one-third of an hour. Setting the pump at 300 milliters per hour will allow 100 milliliters to infuse in the first 20 minutes, and the pump will then alarm and/or shut down.

2. *Answer:* 63 milliters per hour

   Solution: 500 ml = 8 hr = 62.5 = 63 ml/hr

   Rationale: Sixty-three milliliters per hour will deliver 500 milliliters every 8 hours.

3. *Answer:* 125 milliliters per hour

   Solution: 3000 ml ÷ 24 hr = 125 ml/hr

   Rationale: The total intravenous fluid ordered is 3000 milliliters, which 125 milliliters per hour will deliver in 24 hours.

4. *Answer:* 217 milliliters per hour

   Solution: 650 ml ÷ 3 hr = 217 ml/hr

   Rationale: A rate of 217 milliliters per hour will deliver 650 milliliters in 3 hours.

5. *Answer:* 200 milliliters per hour

   Solution: 1000 ml ÷ 5 hr = 200 ml/hr

   Rationale: The period from 9 am to 2 pm is a total of 5 hours. Therefore, 200 milliliters per hour will deliver 1000 milliliters over a 5-hour period.

Answers to Practice Questions for Calculating Drops per Minute

1. *Answers:* 125 ml/hr and 21 gtts/min

   Solution: 1000 ml ÷ 8 hours = 125 ml/hr

   $$\frac{125\,\text{ml}}{60\,\text{min}} \times \frac{10}{1} = 20.8 = 21\,\text{gtts/min}$$

   Rationale: The first step is to determine the milliliters per hour to be infused, reducing to the smallest numbers possible (i.e., numbers reduced to their lowest terms). The larger the number, the greater the chance of a calculation error. The next step is to calculate the gtts/min using the formula.

2. *Answer:* 133 gtts/min

   $$\text{Solution:}\ \frac{100\,\text{ml}}{15\,\text{min}} \times \frac{20}{1} = 133.3 = 133\,\text{gtts/min}$$

   Rationale: There is no reason to calculate the milliliters per hour because the solution will run in 15 minutes. Just calculate the gtts/min using the equation.

3. *Answers:* 150 ml/hr and 38 gtts/min

   $$\text{Solution for gtts/min:}\ \frac{1500\,\text{ml}}{10\,\text{hr}} \times \frac{15}{60} = 37.5 = 38\,\text{gtts/min}$$

   OR

   $$\frac{1500\,\text{ml}}{600\,\text{min}} \times \frac{15}{1} = 37.5 = 38\,\text{gtts/min}$$

Rationale: The 60 is present in the first solution to change the 10 hours into minutes. Remember that the answer to this formula is in drops per minute.

$$\text{Solution for ml/hr:}\ \frac{1500\ \text{ml}}{10\ \text{hr}} = 150\ \text{ml/hr}$$

Rationale: Again, using numbers that are reduced to the lowest terms is always advisable. It is recommended to calculate first the milliliters per hour and then the gtts/min; making the calculations in that order reduces the chances of a calculation error.

4. *Answers:* 167 ml/hr and 167 gtts/min

$$\text{Solution:}\ \frac{2000\ \text{ml}}{12\ \text{hr}} = 166.6 = 167\ \text{ml/hr}$$

$$\frac{167\ \text{ml}}{60\ \text{min}} \times \frac{60}{1} = 167\ \text{gtts/min}$$

Rationale: The equivalent of 2 liters is 2000 milliliters to be infused over 12 hours.

5. *Answer:* 50 gtts/min

$$\text{Solution:}\ \frac{75\ \text{ml}}{30\ \text{min}} \times \frac{20}{1} = 50\ \text{gtts/min}$$

Rationale: There is no need to calculate the milliliters per hour because the problem is already in minutes.

Answers to Practice Questions for Calculating Intravenous Infusions with Added Medication

1. *Answers:* 50 ml/hr and 50 gtts/min

   Solution: Using ratio and proportion:

   $$\frac{100\ \text{units}}{500\ \text{ml}} \times \frac{10\ \text{units}}{x\ \text{ml}}$$

   $100x \times 5000$

   $x = 50\ \text{ml/hr}$

   Now that you know you must give 50 ml/hr to deliver 10 units of regular insulin an hour, solve for gtts/min:

   $$\frac{50\ \text{ml}}{1\ \text{hr}} \times \frac{60}{60} = 50\ \text{gtts/min}$$

   Rationale: You must convert the insulin units to milliliters in order to infuse the correct amount of IV fluids.

2. *Answers:* 100 ml/hr and 33 gtts/min

   Solution: Using ratio and proportion:

   1,000,000 units : 1000 ml :: 100,000 units : x ml

   $1,000,000x = 100,000,000$

   $x = 100\ \text{ml/hr}$

Now that you know that you must give 100 ml/hr to deliver 100,000 units of Pen VK an hour, solve for gtts/min:

$$\frac{100\ ml}{1\ hr} \times \frac{20}{60} = \frac{100}{3} = 33\ gtts/min$$

Rationale: Converting units into milliliters is the first step in calculating the milliliters per hour and drops per minute.

Answers to Posttest

1. 167 gtts/min
2. 21 gtts/min
3. 63 gtts/min
4. 150 gtts/min
5. 42 gtts/min
6. 125 ml/hr
7. 188 ml/hr
8. 500 ml/hr
9. 150 ml/hr
10. 167 ml/hr

11. 94 ml/hr and 94 gtts/min
12. 167 ml/hr and 42 gtts/min
13. 125 ml/hr and 21 gtts/min
14. 42 ml/hr and 14 gtts/min
15. 200 ml/hr and 200 gtts/min
16. 100 ml/hr and 17 gtts/min
17. 75 ml/hr and 19 gtts/min
18. 125 ml/hr and 125 gtts/min
19. 42 ml/hr and 11 gtts/min
20. 200 ml/hr and 200 gtts/min

21. *Answers:* 100 ml/hr and 25 gtts/min
Solution: 40 mEq : 1000 ml :: 4 mEq : *x* ml
22. *Answers:* 40 ml/hr and 10 gtts/min
Solution: 1000 mg (1 gm) : 400 ml :: 100 mg : *x* ml
23. *Answers:* 100 ml/hr and 100 gtts/min
Solution: 500 mg : 100 ml :: 500 mg : *x* ml
24. *Answers:* 25 ml/hr and 25 gtts/min
Solution: 60 mg (1 grain) : 500 ml :: 3 mg : *x* ml
25. *Answers:* 150 ml/hr and 25 gtts/min
Solution: 1000 mg (1 gram) : 1000 ml :: 150 mg : *x* ml

Reference

Potter, A. P., & Perry, A. G.. (2005). *Fundamentals of nursing.* St. Louis, MO: Mosby.

7 Calculating Adult Dosages

Introduction

Calculating safe drug doses is critical to the effectiveness of the medication, not to mention its safety. Very often this is done using the client's stature or build as a basis for dosing. In this chapter, you will learn how to calculate safe drug dosages for adults by means of the:

- Body weight method
- Body surface area (BSA) method

Body Weight Method for Calculating Safe Drug Dosages for Adults

Although not used frequently, the body weight method for calculating safe dosages for adults is important for safe medication administration for many clients with cancer, cardiac, and renal difficulties. Often the dosages of the medications used in the treatment of these diseases must be calculated precisely. One way to achieve the required precision is to calculate the client's body weight in relation to the dosage ordered. To do so, take the following steps.

Step 1

Convert the client's weight in pounds (lb) to kilograms (kg). You must know that 16 ounces equals 1 pound and that 2.2 pounds equals 1 kilogram.

■ EXAMPLE:

A client weighs 147 pounds. Divide 147 by 2.2 to determine that the client weighs 66.8 kilograms. ■

Step 2

Calculate the recommended safe dosage in milligrams per kilogram.

■ EXAMPLE:

If the safe dosage of a medication is 10 milligrams per kilogram, multiply 10 milligrams by 66.8 kilograms. The client would be safe with a dose of up to 668 milligrams. ■

Step 3

Compare the recommended safe dosage with the ordered dosage. If the dosage is within the safe guidelines, the medication may be administered as ordered. If, however, the ordered dosage is in excess of the safe guidelines, then the medication should be withheld and the ordering physician notified.

▪ **EXAMPLE:**

If the physician has ordered any dosage up to 668 milligrams, the medication may be administered as ordered. If the prescribed dosage exceeds this amount, do not administer it, and notify the prescribing physician.   ▪

Here are a couple of other points to remember:

- Consider the minimum to maximum safe dosage range. That is, the range between the smallest therapeutic dose to the largest therapeutic dose.
- Check to see whether the dosage ordered is daily, ordered in multiple doses, or a single one-time order.

Step 4

If the dosage is safe, prepare (pour) the individual dosage and proceed to medicate the client. If the calculations indicate that the dosage is prescribed at an unsafe level, withhold the medication and call the doctor.

Example Problems for Calculating by the Body Weight Method

Remember to show all work and to proof all answers.

1. *Information:* The client weighs 116 lb.

   The order is for daptomycin IVPB 200 mg in 100 ml NS over a 30-min period every morning.

   The drop factor on the tubing is 20 gtts/ml.

   The safe dosage range is 4 mg/kg/day.

   The supply is 500 mg in a 10-ml vial.

   Can the dosage be safely administered?

   Calculate:

   The number of kilograms the client weighs: _____ kg

   How much to add to the IV solution: _____ ml of daptomycin.

   The rate of administration: _____ gtts/min; _____ ml/hr

   Is the dosage safe to administer? _____

M *edication Administration Tip*

> Daptomycin is an antibiotic used in the treatment of skin and skin structure infections.

Solution:
The number of kilograms the client weighs:

$$\frac{116\,\text{lb}}{2.2\,\text{kg}} = 52.7\,\text{kg}$$

How much to add to the IV solution:

$$\frac{10 \text{ ml}}{500 \text{ mg}} \times \frac{200 \text{ mg}}{1} = 4 \text{ ml}$$

Add 4 ml to the infusion.

The rate of administration: Given 100 ml in 30 min with a drop factor of 20, the rate should be 67 gtts/min, and set the pump at a rate of 200 ml/hr.

Is the dosage safe to administer? Yes, it is.

52.7 kg × 4 mg/kg/day = 210.8 mg/day

The client may have up to 210.8 mg/day.

2. *Information:* A client weighs 160 lb.

The client has an order for ibutilide fumarate 0.5 mg in 50 ml NS to infuse over a 10-min period.

The drop factor for the tubing is 10 gtts/ml.

The safe dosage range is 0.01 mg/kg.

The supply is 5 mg in a 2-ml vial.

Calculate:

The number of kg the client weighs: _____ kg

How much to add to the IV solution: _____ ml of Ibutilide fumarate

The rate of administration: _____ gtts/min; _____ ml/hr

Is the dosage safe to administer? _____

M edication Administration Tip

> Ibutilide fumarate is an antiarrhythmic used to treat atrial fibrillation or atrial flutter.

Solution:
The number of kilograms the client weighs:

$$\frac{160 \text{ lb}}{2.2 \text{ kg}} = 72.7 \text{ kg}$$

How much to add to the IV solution:

$$\frac{2 \text{ ml}}{5 \text{ mg}} \times \frac{0.5 \text{ mg}}{1} = 0.2 \text{ ml}$$

Add 0.2 ml to the infusion.

The rate of administration: Given 50 ml in 10 min with a drop factor of 10, the rate should be 50 gtts/min, and set the pump at a rate of 300 ml/hr.

Is the dosage safe to administer? Yes, it is.

72.7 kg × 0.01 mg/kg = 7.27 mg

The client may have up to 7.27 mg.

3. *Information:* A client is obese and weighs 320 lb.

The client has an order for mercaptopurine 100 mg po daily.

The safe dosage range is 2.5 mg/kg/day.

The supply consists of 50-mg tablets.

Calculate:

The number of kilograms the client weighs: _____ kg

How much to administer: _____ tablets

Is the dosage safe to administer? _____

M edication Administration Tip

> Mercaptopurine is an antineoplastic antimetabolite used to treat acute lympho-cytic or myelocytic leukemia.

Solution:
The number of kilograms the client weighs:

$$\frac{320\,lb}{2.2\,kg} = 145.4\,kg$$

How much to administer:

$$\frac{1\,tablet}{50\,mg} \times \frac{100\,mg}{1} = 2\,tablets$$

Is the dosage safe to administer? Yes, it is.

145.5 kg × 2.5 mg/kg/day = 362.5 mg/day

The client may take up to 362.5 mg per day.

Body Surface Area (BSA) Method for Calculating Safe Drug Dosages for Adults

The body surface area method, also not used very frequently, nevertheless plays an important role when calculating potent drugs, such as chemotherapy agents and certain cardiac and renal medications. BSA calculations are based on the client's height and weight, and the solution is expressed in square meters (m²). Charts, known as nomograms, are also available, and solutions are calculated for you. See Figure 7-1. Remember, though, that the nurse or healthcare provider is responsible for determining, based on BSA, whether the ordered dosage is safe to give.

Body Surface Area Formulas

There are two options when calculating the client's BSA. One uses the metric system, and the other uses the household measurement system. Both use the same formula.

FIGURE 7-1 Adult body surface area nomogram.

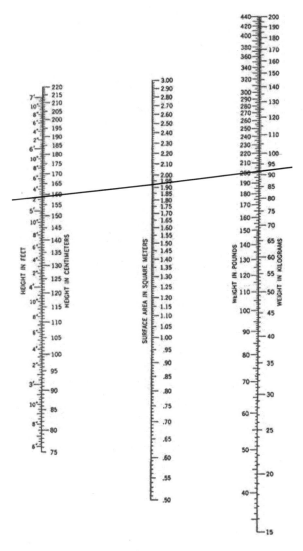

To calculate an adult's BSA, draw a straight line from the height (left column) to the weight (right column). The point at which the line intersects the surface area column is the BSA.

Option 1

- Convert the client's height (in feet and inches) to centimeters. (Remember that 1 inch equals 2.5 centimeters and that 1 foot equals 30 centimeters.)
- Convert the client's weight (in pounds and ounces) to kilograms. (Remember that 2.2 pounds equals 1 kilogram.)
- Then apply the following formula:

$$\text{BSA (m}^2) = \sqrt{\frac{\text{Height (cm)} \times \text{Weight (kg)}}{3600}}$$

Option 2

In the household system of measurement, use the client's height in inches (1 foot equals 12 inches) and the client's weight in pounds and ounces (16 ounces equals 1 pound). Then apply the following formula:

$$\text{BSA (m}^2) = \sqrt{\frac{\text{Height (in)} \times \text{Weight (lb)}}{3131}}$$

Practice Questions for Calculating a Client's Height and Weight

Fill in the blanks with the missing information. Remember to show all work and to proof all answers.

1. Client's weight: 95.4 kg = _____ lb

2. Client's height: 5 ft 4 in = _____ in = _____ cm

3. Client's weight: 180 lb = _____ kg

4. Client's height: 71 in = _____ cm

5. Client's weight: 120 lb = _____ kg

6. Client's height: 5 ft 2 in = _____ in = _____ cm

7. Client's weight: 61.3 kg = _____ lb

8. Client's height: 5 ft 6 in = _____ in = _____ cm

9. Client's weight: 190 lb = _____ kg

10. Client's height: 6 ft 2 in = _____ in = _____ cm

Practice Questions for Calculating Safe Client Dosages Using Body Weight and Body Surface Area Methods

Remember to show all work and to proof all answers.

1. *Information:* The client weighs 140 lb and is 5 ft 6 in tall.

The doctor orders abatacept (Orencia) 500 mg intravenously in 250 ml NS to infuse over 1 hr as a one-time dose.

The safe dosage range is as follows:

      <60 kg = 500 mg every 2 weeks × 3 doses

      60–100 kg = 750 mg every 2 weeks × 3 doses

The supply is 250 mg per 15-ml vial.

Calculate:

140 lb = _____ kg

5 ft 6 in = _____ in = _____ cm

Apply the body weight method (BWM):

_____

Give: _____

Is the dosage safe? _____

M edication Administration Tip

> Abatacept is an antirheumatic used to treat the signs and symptoms and the progression of rheumatoid arthritis.

2. *Information:* The client is 6 ft 0 in tall and weighs 250 lb.

   The MD orders agalsidase beta (Fabrazyme) 150 mg IVPB X one dose.

   The safe dosage range is 1 mg/kg every 2 weeks.

   The supply is 5 mg/1 ml in 20-ml vials.

   Calculate:

   250 lb = _____ kg

   6 ft 0 in = _____ in = _____ cm

   Apply the body weight method:

   _____

   Give: _____

   Is the dosage safe? _____

M edication Administration Tip

> Agalsidase beta is a replacement enzyme used to treat clients with Fabry disease.

3. *Information:* The client weighs 115 lb and is 5 ft 2 in tall.

   The physician orders panitumumab (Vectibix) 250 mg IVPB to infuse over 60 min every 2 weeks.

   The safe dosage range is 6 mg/kg every 2 weeks.

   The supply is 20 mg/ml in 5-ml vials.

   Calculate:

   115 lb = _____ kg

   5 ft 2 in = _____ in = _____ cm

   Apply the body weight method:

   _____

   Give: _____

   Is the dosage safe? _____

M edication Administration Tip

> Panitumumab is an antineoplastic agent used to treat metastatic colorectal cancer.

4. *Information:* The client weighs 125 lb and stands 5 ft 7 in tall.

Nelarabine (Arranon) 250 mg is ordered by the doctor to be given IVPB 3 times a week for 1 week.

The safe dosage range is 1500 mg/m^2 3 times a week for 1 week.

The supply is 5 mg/1 ml in 50-ml vials.

Calculate:

125 lb = _____ kg

5 ft 7 in = _____ in = _____ cm

Apply the body surface area (BSA) method:

_____

Give: _____

Is the dosage safe? _____

M edication Administration Tip

> Nelarabine is an antineoplastic agent used in the treatment of T-cell acute lymphoblastic leukemia.

5. *Information:* The client weighs 180 lb and is 5 ft 8 in tall.

Deferasirox (Exjade) is ordered for a client after receiving 2 units of packed red blood cells. The client is to take 500 mg po every morning.

The safe dosage range is 20 mg/kg/day.

The supply is 250-mg tablets.

Calculate:

180 lb = _____ kg

5 ft 8 in = _____ in = _____ cm

Apply the body weight method:

_____

Give: _____

Is the dosage safe? _____

M *edication Administration Tip*

> Deferasirox is a chelating agent used in the treatment of iron (Fe) overload for clients receiving multiple blood transfusions.

POSTTEST

Fill in the blanks with the missing information. Remember to show all work and to proof all answers.

1. Calcium EDTA is ordered for a client with a BSA of 1.70 m².

   The safe dosage range for this medication is 250 mg/m².

   How much calcium EDTA should the healthcare provider administer? _____ mg

2. A client diagnosed with metastatic lung cancer has Oncovin solution (vincristine) 3 mg IV ordered. The client's BSA is 1.7 m².

   The safe dosage range for this medication is 2 mg/m².

   The supply is 1 mg per 1 ml.

   How much solution should the nurse prepare to administer? _____ ml

   Is the ordered dosage safe to give? _____.

Find the BSA for the following clients, using the nomogram in Figure 7-1.

3. A client who is 5 ft 1 in tall and weighs 130 lb is _____ m².

4. An obese client who stands 5 ft 4 in and has a weight of 180 lb is _____ m².

5. A client 5 ft 5 in in height and 160 lb in weight is _____ m².

Answer questions 6–10 based on the following scenario using the body weight method.

   A client has an order for 100 mg gentamicin IVPB every 8 hr (300 mg every 24 hr). The client weighs 176 lb and is 5 ft 8 in tall.

   The safe dosage range for this medication is up to 1.7 mg/kg/IV every 8 hr.

   The supply is 80 mg/2 ml.

6. The client weighs _____ kg.

7. The client's height is _____ cm.

8. What is the maximum dosage of gentamicin this client may receive once every 8 hr? _____ mg

9. What is the maximum dosage of gentamicin that the client may receive every 24 hr? _____ mg

10. Is the dosage ordered for this client within the safe range? _____ Explain your answer.

_____

_____

_____

Answer questions 11–20 using the nomogram in Figure 7-1. Calculate the BSA for the following clients:

11. Height: 6 ft 2 in; weight: 260 lb; BSA: _____

12. Height: 5 ft 0 in; weight: 110 lb; BSA: _____

13. Height: 5 ft 8 in; weight: 210 lb; BSA: _____

14. Height: 5 ft 10 in; weight: 185 lb; BSA: _____

15. Height: 6 ft 0 in; weight: 165 lb; BSA: _____

16. Height: 170 cm; weight: 40 kg; BSA: _____

17. Height: 190 cm; weight: 60 kg; BSA: _____

18. Height: 220 cm; weight: 55 kg; BSA: _____

19. Height: 155 cm; weight: 80 kg; BSA: _____

20. Height: 185 cm; weight: 72 kg; BSA: _____

Answers

Answers to Practice Questions for Calculating a Client's Height and Weight

1. 210 lb
2. 64 in; 160 cm
3. 82 kg
4. 177.5 cm
5. 54 kg
6. 62 in; 155 cm
7. 135 lbs
8. 66 in; 165 cm
9. 86 kg
10. 74 in; 185 cm

Answers to Practice Questions for Calculating Safe Client Dosages Using Body Weight and Body Surface Area Methods

1. 63.6 kg

   66 in; 165 cm

   $$\frac{750 \text{ mg}}{60 \text{ kg}} \times 63.6 \text{ kg} = 795 \text{ mg/dose}$$

   Give: 30 ml

   Yes, the dosage is safe.

2. 113.6 kg

   72 in; 180 cm

   $$\frac{1 \text{ mg}}{1 \text{ kg}} \times 113.6 \text{ kg} = 114 \text{ (rounded) mg}$$

   Give: 30 ml

   No, the dosage is not safe.

3. 52.2 kg

   62 in; 155 cm

   $$\frac{6 \text{ mg}}{1 \text{ kg}} \times 52.2 \text{ kg} = 313.2 \text{ mg}$$

   Give: 62.5 ml

   Yes, the dosage is safe.

4. 56.8 kg

   67 in; 167.5 cm

   $$\sqrt{\frac{167.5 \text{ cm} \times 56.8 \text{ kg}}{3600}} = 1.62 \text{ m}^2$$

   Give: 50 ml or 1 vial

   Yes, the dosage is safe.

5. 81.8 kg

   68 in; 170 cm

   $$\frac{20 \text{ mg}}{1 \text{ kg}} \times 81.8 \text{ kg} = 1636 \text{ mg}$$

   Give: 2 tablets

   Yes, the dosage is safe.

Answers to Posttest

1. 425 mg ($1.70 \text{ m}^2 \times 250 \text{ mg/m}^2$)

2. How much solution to prepare:

   $$\frac{1 \text{ mg}}{1 \text{ ml}} \times \frac{3 \text{ mg}}{1} = 3 \text{ ml}$$

   Yes, the dosage is safe (safe range: $1.70 \text{ m}^2 \times 2 \text{ mg/m}^2 = 3.40 \text{ mg}$).

3. 1.59 m^2

4. 1.92 m^2

5. 1.82 m^2

6. 80 kg

7. 170 cm

8. 136 mg

   $$\frac{1.7 \text{ mg/8 hr}}{1 \text{ kg}} \times 80 \text{ kg} = 136 \text{ mg}$$

9. 408 mg (136 mg × 3 8-hr periods/24 hr)

10. Yes, the dosage is safe. The dose to be given every 8 hr (100 mg) is less than the maximum 8-hr dose (136 mg), and the 24-hr dose to be given (300 mg) is less than the maximum total 24-hr dose (408 mg).

11. 2.43 m^2

12. 1.45 m^2

13. 2.09 m^2

14. 1.81 m^2

15. 1.96 m^2

16. 1.43 m^2

17. 1.84 m^2

18. 1.97 m^2

19. 1.79 m^2

20. 1.95 m^2

8 Pediatric Dosages and Medicating Children

Introduction

Accuracy and precision are paramount when medicating pediatric clients. The most precise methods for calculating pediatric dosages are

- Calculating the client's body weight in kilograms, known as the body weight method.
- Calculating the client's body surface area (BSA) in square meters.

This chapter guides you in:

- Applying both the body weight and the BSA methods, the latter using a nomogram for infants and children (see Figure 8-1).
- Employing appropriate techniques when medicating infants and children of various ages.
- Making the appropriate calculations in administering intravenous pediatric fluids.

Body Weight Method for Calculating Safe Drug Dosages in the Pediatric Client

Often the dosage of the medications used in the treatment of pediatric diseases must be calculated precisely. One way to accomplish the required precision is to calculate the child's body weight in relation to the dosage ordered. To apply the body weight method to pediatric clients, follow these steps.

Step 1

Convert the child's weight in pounds (lb) to kilograms (kg). Remember that 16 ounces equals 1 pound and 2.2 pounds = 1 kilogram.

M edication Administration Tip

> Factors to consider when calculating pediatric medication dosages include the child's age, weight, body surface area, and the amount of the medication (Potter & Perry, 2005, p. 837).

EXAMPLE:

A child weighs 47 pounds. Divide this weight by 2.2 to determine that the child weighs 21.3 kilograms.

Step 2

Calculate the recommended safe dosage range in milligrams per kilogram.

FIGURE 8-1 Nomogram for estimating the surface area of infants and children.

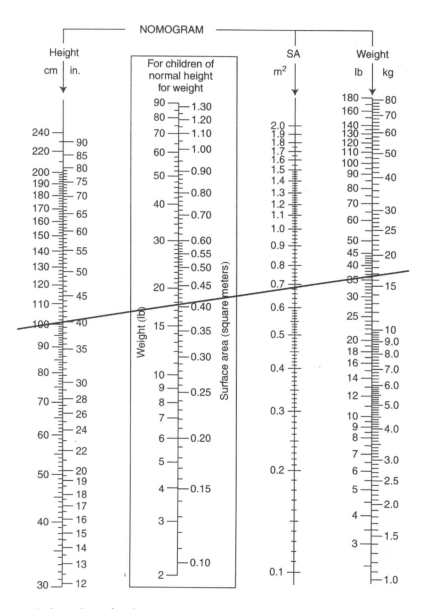

Pediatric doses of medications are generally based on body surface area (BSA) or weight. To calculate a child's BSA, draw a straight line from the height (in the left-hand column) to the weight (in the right-hand column). The point at which the line intersects the surface area (SA) column is the BSA (measured in square meters [m²]). If the child is of roughly normal proportion, BSA can be calculated from the weight alone (in the enclosed area).

Source: Modified from data of E. Boyd by C. D. West; from Behrman, R. E., Kliegman, R. M., & Jenson, H. B. (Eds.). (2000). *Nelson textbook of pediatrics* (16th ed.). Philadelphia: W. B. Saunders.

■ **EXAMPLE:**

If the safe dosage of a medication is 10 milligrams per kilogram, multiply 10 milligrams by 21.3 kilograms. The child would be safe with a dose of up to 213 mg. ■

Step 3

Compare the recommended safe dosage range with the ordered dosage. If the dosage is within the safe guidelines, the medication may be administered as ordered. If, however, the ordered dosage is in excess of the safe guidelines, then the medication should be held and the ordering physician notified.

■ **EXAMPLE:**

If the dosage ordered is less than 213 milligrams, it may be administered. If it is more than 213 milligrams, notify the physician. ■

Here are some other important points to remember when calculating the safety range for pediatric clients:

- Consider the minimum to maximum safe dosage range.
- Check to see whether the dosage is daily, in multiple doses, or a single one-time order.
- Most medications on the market today that are used for pediatric clients are labeled with the safe dosage range for children based on milligrams per kilogram. Many of these medications also list the safe dosing range for adults, which you can use to check your pediatric dosage calculations. For example, if the safe dosing range for an average adult is 10 milligrams per kilogram and you determine that your pediatric safe dosing range is 15 milligrams per kilogram, pause and think. Is the safe pediatric dosing range really likely to be greater than the safe adult dosing range? Of course, it is not. You should recalculate and proof your answer.

Step 4

If the dosage is safe, prepare the individual dosage and proceed to medicate the child. If the calculations demonstrate an unsafe level, withhold the medication and call the doctor.

Practice Questions for Calculating by the Body Weight Method for Pediatric Clients

Remember to show all work and to proof all answers.

1. An 8-year-old child weighs 40 lb. The child has an order for mecasermin (Increlex) 1 mg subcutaneously BID. The safe dosage range is up to 0.08 mg/kg BID. The supply is 10 mg/ml in 4-ml vials.

   Calculate:

   40 lb = _____ kg

   The maximum safe dosage range for this child is _____ mg BID.

   The number of milliliters you will administer for one dose is _____ ml.

   Is the dosage safe to administer? _____

M edication Administration Tip

> Mecasermin is a growth hormone used in the long-term treatment of growth failure due to growth factor-1.

2. An infant who weighs 16 lb is ordered to have ibuprofen lysine 35 mg intravenously at 8 am today and tomorrow. The safe dosing range for this medication is 5 mg/kg × 2 doses given 24 hr apart. The supply for the medication is 10 mg/ml in 2-ml vials.

Calculate:

16 lb = _____ kg

The safe dosage range for this infant is _____ mg × 2 doses 24 hr apart.

The number of milliliters you will administer for one dose is _____ ml.

Is the dosage safe? _____

M edication Administration Tip

> Ibuprofen lysine is a nonsteroidal anti-inflammatory agent used in the treatment of patent ductus arteriosus (PDA).

3. A 15-month-old toddler, weighing 22 lb, is ordered to receive alglucosidase 100 mg intravenously every 2 weeks. The safe dosing range is 20 mg/kg every 2 weeks. The supply is 50 mg/20-ml vial.
   Calculate:

22 lb = _____ kg

The safe dosage range for this toddler is _____ mg once every 2 weeks.

The number of milliliters you will administer for one dose is _____ ml.

Is the dosage safe? _____

M edication Administration Tip

> Alglucosidase is a replacement hormone used in the treatment of Pompe disease.

Body Surface Area (BSA) Method for Calculating Safe Drug Dosages in the Pediatric Client

The body surface area (BSA) method for calculating safe drug dosages is also used very frequently in calculating pediatric dosages. BSA calculations require reconfiguring the child's height and weight and expressing them in terms of square meters (m^2). Charts, known as nomograms, are also available, and the solutions are calculated for you (see Figure 8-1). Remember, though, that the nurse or healthcare provider is responsible for determining whether the ordered dosage is safe to give.

Body Surface Area Formulas

Just as when the BSA method is applied to adults, there are two options to choose from when calculating the pediatric client's BSA. The following is a review from Chapter 7.

Option 1

- Convert the child's height (in feet and inches) to centimeters. (Remember that 1 inch equals 2.5 centimeters and that 1 foot equals 30 centimeters.)
- Convert the child's weight (in pounds and ounces) to kilograms. (Remember that 2.2 pounds equals 1 kilogram.)

1. $\text{BSA (m}^2) = \sqrt{\dfrac{\text{Height (cm)} \times \text{Weight (kg)}}{3600}}$

Option 2

In the household system of measurement, use the child's height in inches (1 foot equals 12 inches) and the child's weight in pounds (16 ounces equals 1 pound). Then apply the following formula:

2. $\text{BSA (m}^2) = \sqrt{\dfrac{\text{Height (in)} \times \text{Weight (lb)}}{3131}}$

Practice Questions for Calculating a Pediatric Client's Height and Weight

Fill in the blanks with the missing information. Remember to show all work and to proof all answers.

1. Child's weight: 9 kg = _____ lb
2. Child's height: 3 ft 4 in = _____ in = _____ cm
3. Child's weight: 32 lb = _____ kg

Medicating the Pediatric Client

Because medicating pediatric clients can often be problematic, having the parents assist is helpful. There are many ways to prepare a child emotionally and physically for taking medications. Potter and Perry (2005) offer the following useful suggestions:

- Offer liquids rather than pills. Liquids are easier and safer for the child to swallow.
- Use medication droppers for infants and straws for older children to help swallowing.
- Offer a flavored juice or an ice pop afterward to relieve aftertaste.
- If a mixture of medications and fluids is called for, use the smallest amount possible.
- Do not mix medications with the child's favorite food items. The association may cause them to refuse to eat the food in the future.
- Have someone (preferably a parent) restrain a child when necessary to avoid doing harm.
- Never inject a sleeping child. The child should first be awakened.
- Use distraction when injecting a child, such as toys, pictures, or sounds, to reduce the child's perception of pain.
- Apply a local anesthetic to the skin before injecting whenever possible.

Intravenous Pediatric Fluid Administration

Pediatric clients receive intravenous fluids through the use of volume control sets (see Figure 8-2), which administers a prescribed amount of fluid on an hourly basis. The chamber is filled with small amounts of fluids to be administered while the upper tubing is clamped off to prevent an infant or child from receiving too much fluid. The chamber is filled every hour and typically can hold up to 100–150 milliliters of fluid. Medication may also be added to the fluid volume chamber, if it is ordered. The drop factor on the fluid volume chamber is usually 60 gtts/ml.

The formulas for calculating pediatric intravenous fluid administration are the same as explained in Chapter 6.

The two formulas for calculating drops per minute are

$$\frac{\text{Total volume (TV)}}{\text{Total time (TT, in hours)}} \times \frac{\text{Drop factor}}{60 \text{ minutes}} = \text{Drops per minute}$$

$$\frac{\text{Total volume (TV)}}{\text{Total time (TT, in minutes)}} \times \frac{\text{Drop factor}}{1} = \text{Drops per minute}$$

To calculate the milliliters per hour, use the following formula:

$$\frac{\text{Total volume}}{\text{Total time (hr)}} = \text{Infusion rate per hour (ml/hr)}$$

FIGURE 8-2 Pediatric fluid volume control set.

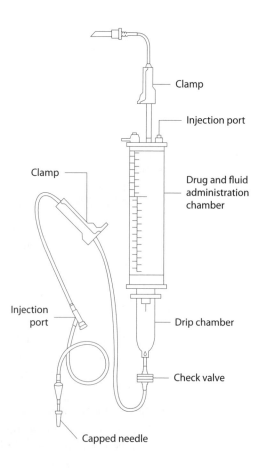

Practice Questions for Pediatric Intravenous Fluid Administration

Remember to show all work and to proof all answers.

1. The physician orders 50 ml/hr of D5NS for a child using a pediatric volume control set. The nurse fills the volume chamber with 100 ml of fluid and sets the infusion pump.

   Calculate:

   How long will it take the volume chamber to empty? _____

   How many gtts per minute should there be? _____

   At how many milliliters per hour should the infusion pump be set? _____ ml/hr

2. A child has an intravenous infusion running at 30 ml/hr. The pediatrician orders gentamicin 20 mg IV to run in 30 min. The supply of the medication is 40 mg/2 ml. The nurse fills the volume chamber and sets the infusion pump.

   Calculate:

   How much gentamicin should be placed in the volume chamber? _____ ml

   How much intravenous fluid should be placed in the volume chamber? _____ ml for a total of _____ ml

   How long should it take to administer the gentamicin? _____

3. For a child, the physician orders 35 ml/hr of D5W using a pediatric volume control set. The nurse fills the volume chamber with 100 ml of fluid and sets the infusion pump.

   Calculate:

   How long will it take the volume chamber to empty? _____

   How many gtts per minute should there be? _____

   At how many milliliters per hour should the infusion pump should be set? _____ ml/hr

4. The child has an intravenous infusion running at 60 ml/hr. The pediatrician orders Lasix (furosemide) 80 mg IV to run in 20 min. The supply of the medication is 20 mg/2 ml. The nurse fills the volume chamber and sets the infusion pump.

   Calculate:

   How much Lasix should be placed in the volume chamber? _____ ml

   How much intravenous fluid should be placed in the volume chamber? _____ ml for a total of _____ ml

   How long should it take to administer the Lasix? _____

POSTTEST

Remember to show all work and to proof all answers.
For questions 1–5, refer to the nomogram in Figure 8-1.

1. 10 lb and 23 in = _____ m^2
2. 18 lb and 26 in = _____ m^2
3. 7 lb and 20 in = _____ m^2
4. 30 lb and 40 in = _____ m^2
5. 35 kg and 55 cm = _____ m^2

For questions 6–10, fill in the missing information.

6. 35 lb = _____ kg
7. 12 kg = _____ lb
8. 8 lb 3 oz = _____ kg
9. 3.2 kg = _____ lb
10. 21 lb = _____ kg

For questions 11–15, read the word problems and make the required calculations.

11. A toddler weighs 22 lb and is to have the safe dosage range of an antibiotic medication every 12 hr. The safe dosage range is 20 mg/kg/day in divided doses. The supply is 100 mg/5 ml.

    Calculate:

    22 lb = _____ kg

    The safe dosage limit per day is _____ ml or _____ mg.

    Give: _____ ml every 12 hr

12. A child weighs 35 lb and is ordered to take 0.5 mg of a medication po every morning. The safe dosage range is 0.1 mg/kg/day in divided doses. The supply is 0.1 mg/1 ml in a 5-ml vial.

    Calculate:

    35 lb = _____ kg

    The safe dosage limit per day is _____ ml or _____ mg.

    Give: _____ ml every morning

13. An infant weighs 10 lb 8 oz and needs 5 mg of a medication BID. The safe dosage range is 2 mg/kg/day. The supply is 1 mg/1 ml oral suspension.

    Calculate:

    10 lb 8 oz = _____ kg

    The safe dosage limit per day is _____ ml or _____ mg.

    Give: _____ ml BID

14. A child weighs 80 lb and is to have 100 mg of an antibiotic every 6 hr IVPB. The safe dosage range is 15 mg/kg/day in divided doses. The supply is 50 mg/10 ml.

    Calculate:

80 lb = _____ kg

The safe dosage limit per day is _____ ml or _____ mg.

Give: _____ ml IVPB every 6 hr.

15. A 2-year-old child weighs 40 lb. He is to have 30 mg of a medication TID. The safe dosage range is 5 mg/kg/day. The supply is 125 mg/5 ml.

Calculate:

40 lb = _____ kg

The safe dosage limit per day is _____ ml or _____ mg.

Give: _____ ml TID

M edication Administration Tip

Tylenol (acetaminophen) is an antipyretic and nonnarcotic analgesic. It is frequently given to children to reduce fevers and alleviate moderate discomforts associated with the common cold, flu, and various viral and bacterial infections. It is available in chewable tablets (80 mg), suppositories (80 mg, 120 mg, 125 mg), liquid (160 mg/5 ml), and sprinkle capsules (80 mg, 160 mg). Pediatric patients may be dosed up to 5 times per day unless otherwise ordered by the physician. The maximum safe dosage for pediatric patients is 1 kg/16 mg/dose. The following is a breakdown of pediatric ages and safe dosages.

Age	Dosage (mg)
–3 mos	40
4–11 mos	80
1–2 yr	120
2–3 yr	160
4–5 yr	240
6–8 yr	320
9–10 yr	400
11 yr	480

For questions 16–25, answer based on the pediatric medication information provided in the following clinical scenario.

Clinical Scenario

A 3-year-old pediatric client weighing 22 lb is brought to the community clinic by his mother with complaints of nausea, vomiting, fever, malaise, and generalized aches and pains. The clinic physician diagnoses the child with a viral infection and discusses with the mother how to treat the symptoms. He orders a clear liquid diet, rest, and Tylenol for the fever and discomfort. The mother tells the doctor that her son is unable to swallow pills and refuses to chew them either.

16. How many kilograms does the child weigh? _____ kg

17. If the child is medicated with Tylenol at 11 am, how much should the mother give? _____ mg

18. What form of Tylenol would be best for this child?
    _____

19. How much liquid Tylenol should the mother prepare to give? _____ ml

20. When will it be safe for the mother to medicate the child a second time, if necessary? _____ pm

21. Name three items the mother should verify on the medication label before preparing and administering the Tylenol.
    a. _____
    b. _____
    c. _____

22. What household utensil should the mother use to administer 5 ml of liquid Tylenol? _____

23. What is the maximum safe dosage of Tylenol that may be administered for a single dose for this child? _____ mg

24. Tylenol is the: (choose the right answer)
    a. Trade name
    b. Generic name
    c. Registry name
    d. Pharmacologic name

25. Acetaminophen is the: (choose the correct answer)
    a. Trade name
    b. Generic name
    c. Registry name
    d. Pharmacologic name

Answers

Answers to Practice Questions for Calculating by the Body Weight Method for Pediatric Clients

1. 18 kg
   1.44 mg
   0.1 ml
   Yes, the dosage is safe.
2. 7.2 kg
   36 mg

   3.5 ml
   Yes, the dosage is safe.
3. 10 kg
   200 mg
   40 ml
   Yes, the dosage is safe.

Answers to Practice Questions for Calculating a Pediatric Client's Height and Weight

1. 19.8 lb
2. 40 in; 100 cm
3. 14.5 kg

Answers to Practice Questions for Pediatric Intravenous Fluid Administration

1. 2 hr
   50 gtts/min
   50 ml/hr
2. 1 ml
   14 ml; 15 ml
   30 min
3. 2.85 hr
   35 gtts/min
   35 ml/hr
4. 8 ml
   12 ml; 20 ml
   20 min

Answers to Posttest

1. 0.27 m^2
2. 0.4 m^2
3. 0.21 m^2
4. 0.61 m^2
5. 0.73 m^2
6. 15 .9 kg
7. 26.4 lb
8. 3.85 kg
9. 7.04 lb
10. 9.5 kg
11. 10 kg
    10 ml; 200 mg
    5 ml every 12 hr
12. 15.9 kg
    15.9 ml; 1.59 mg
    5 ml every morning
13. 4.9 kg
    9.8 ml; 9.8 mg
    5 ml BID
14. 36.3 kg
    109 ml; 545 mg
    20 ml IVPB every 6 hr
15. 18 kg
    3.6 ml; 90 mg
    1.2 ml TID
16. 10 kg
17. 160 mg
18. liquid
19. 5 ml
20. 4 pm
21. Any of the following are correct answers: warnings/alerts, drug name, drug strength, drug route, dosages supplied, expiration date
22. 1 teaspoon
23. 160 mg
24. a
25. b

Reference

Potter, A. P., & Perry, A. G. (2005). *Fundamentals of nursing.* St. Louis, MO: Mosby.

9 Comprehensive Examination I

Unless otherwise instructed, answer the questions by filling in the missing information. Be sure to show all work and to proof all answers.

1. 1000 mg = _____ g

2. The MD orders 1000 ml IV D5RL to infuse in 8 hr. The drop factor on the tubing is 10 gtts/ml.

   Give: _____ gtts/min   _____ ml/hr

3. 60 mg = gr _____

4. The MD orders 500 mg of a medication. On hand is 1 g of the medication in 5 ml. Give: _____

   Solve using the following three methods.

   Ratio and proportion method:

   Dosage formula method:

   Dimensional analysis method:

---

5. A child weighs 30 lb and has an order for ampicillin 50 mg po QID. The safe dosage range for the drug is 15 mg/kg in divided doses. The supply is 50 mg/5 ml oral suspension. *Calculate*:

   30 lb = _____ kg

   Safe dosage limit per day: _____ mg or _____ ml

   Give: _____ ml po QID

6. 1 tsp = _____ gtts

7. 1 qt = _____ ml

8. 1 gtt = _____ minim

9. 8 oz = _____ ml

10. The doctor orders 1000 ml D5W with 40 mEq KCL to run at 2 mEq/hr. The drop factor on the tubing is 20 gtts/ml. *Calculate*:

    _____ gtts/min   _____ ml/hr

11. The nurse practitioner has ordered Benadryl 50 mg IVPB Q6H PRN for itch for a postoperative client. The supply is 10 mg/1 ml in a 10-ml vial. The nurse prepares the IVPB with 100 ml D/NS to run in 20 min. The drop factor on the tubing is 15 gtts/ml. *Calculate*:

    Benadryl 50 mg = _____ ml

    _____ gtts/min   _____ ml/hr

12. 1000 mg = gr _____

For questions 13–17, convert to decimals.

13. $^3/_8$ = _____
14. $^4/_5$ = _____
15. $^1/_2$ = _____
16. $^9/_{10}$ = _____
17. $^3/_{16}$ = _____

For questions 18–20, reduce to the lowest terms.

18. $^9/_{27}$ = _____
19. $^1/_6 + ^3/_6$ = _____
20. $^{36}/_9$ = _____

For questions 21–25, convert to Roman numerals.

21. 1968 = _____
22. 109 = _____
23. 7.5 = _____
24. 650 = _____
25. 444 = _____
26. 3.5 L = _____ ml
27. 500 mg = _____ g
28. 16 oz = _____ pt
29. 2 qt = _____ oz
30. 60 minims = _____ fluidrams
31. 6 mg = gr _____
32. 30 mg = _____ drams
33. 1 kg = _____ lb
34. 454 g = _____ lb
35. 5 ml = _____ minims
36. 60 mg : gr I :: x × mg : gr XX x = _____ mg
37. 15 ml : 1 tbs :: x ml : 6 tbs x = _____ ml

38. $\dfrac{250\ mg}{500\ mg} \times 4\ ml$ = _____ ml

39. $\dfrac{1\ g}{500\ mg} \times 1\ tablet$ = _____ tablets

40. $x\ tablets = \dfrac{1\ tablet}{25\ mg} \times \dfrac{75\ mg}{1}$ = _____ tablets

41. $x \text{ ml} = \dfrac{20 \text{ ml}}{100 \text{ mg}} \times \dfrac{200 \text{ mg}}{1} = \underline{\hspace{2cm}} \text{ ml}$

42. Name the six steps/rights to safely administering medications.

    a.

    b.

    c.

    d.

    e.

    f.

43. The MD orders 250 ml D5NS to infuse in 5 hr. Microtubing is used. *Calculate*:

    _____ gtts/min   _____ ml/hr

44. The MD orders 1000 ml D5W, 1000 ml D5NS, and 1000 ml D5RL to infuse in the next 24 hr. *Calculate*:

    _____ ml/hr

45. The MD orders 1 g of Kefzol in 100 ml NS to be given IVPB over a 30-min period. The drop factor on the tubing is 20 gtts/ml. *Calculate*:

    _____ gtts/min   _____ ml/hr

46. At 9 am a client's IV of D5W has 325 ml left in the bottle (LIB). The physician has ordered the remaining fluid to be infused by noon and the IV discontinued. At what rate should the nurse set the infusion pump?

    _____ ml/hr

47. Height: 6 ft 2 in = _____ in = _____ cm

48. Weight: 210 lb = _____ kg

49. Height: 5 ft 3 in = _____ in = _____ cm

50. Weight: 120 lb = _____ kg

51. The MD orders 30 mg of a medication. The supply consists of gr I scored tablets.

    Give: _____

    Solve using the following three methods.

    Ratio and proportion method:

    Dosage formula method:

    Dimensional analysis method:

52. 15 mg = gr _____

53. The doctor orders an IV of 500 ml NS with 1 ampule of MVI to run in 2 hr. The drop factor on the tubing is 15 gtts/ml. *Calculate*:

    _____ gtts/min   _____ ml/hr

54. The nurse anesthetist orders morphine 15 mg IVPB Q4H PRN for pain for a postoperative client. The supply is 30 mg/ml in a 5-ml vial. The postanesthesia care nurse prepares the IVPB with 50 ml NS to run in 15 min. Microtubing is used. *Calculate*:

    Morphine 15 mg = _____ ml

    _____ gtts/min   _____ ml/hr

55. A client scheduled for discharge has 200 ml of D5RL left in his IV bag at 7 am. He tells you that his wife is picking him up at 9 am. The doctor writes an order

to infuse the remaining fluid and then discontinue the IV line. The drop factor on the tubing is 10 gtts/ml. At what rate should the nurse infuse the fluid?

_____ gtts/min   _____ ml/hr

56. Circle the brand name of the drug on the label provided.

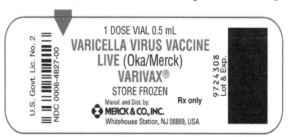

Source: Courtesy of Merck & Co., Inc.

57. Circle the route of the drug on the label provided.

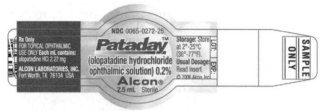

Source: © Alcon Laboratories, Inc. Used with permission.

58. Circle the generic name of the drug on the label provided.

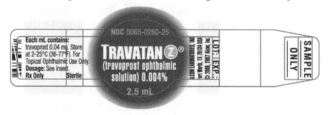

Source: © Alcon Laboratories, Inc. Used with permission.

59. What is the expiration date on the IV bag provided?

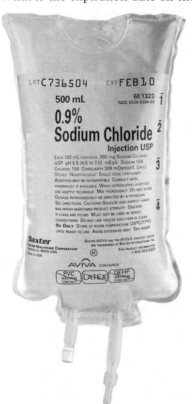

Source: © Baxter Healthcare Corporation. Used with permission.

60. Circle the supply dose of the drug on the label provided.

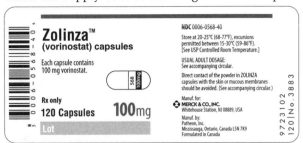

Source: Courtesy of Merck & Co., Inc.

61. Circle the dosage strength of the drug on the label provided.

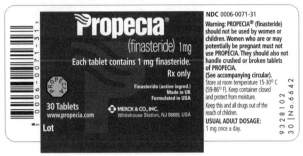

Source: Courtesy of Merck & Co., Inc.

62. Circle the storage directions for the drug on the label provided.

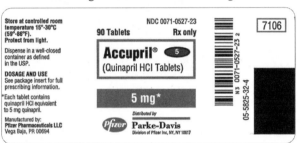

Source: © Pfizer Inc. Used with permission.

63. A patient has Xanax (alprazolam) 0.5 mg ordered. Using the drug label provided, you know to give: _____

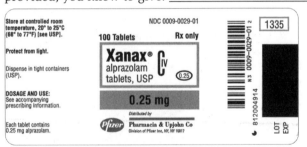

Source: © Pfizer Inc. Used with permission.

64. Circle the number of dosages per container on the label provided.

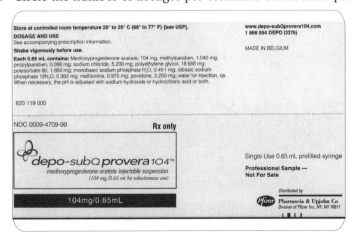

Source: © Pfizer Inc. Used with permission.

65. Circle the directions for the route of the drug on the label provided.

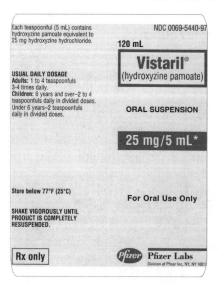

Source: © Pfizer Inc. Used with permission.

66. Circle the trade name of the drug on the label provided.

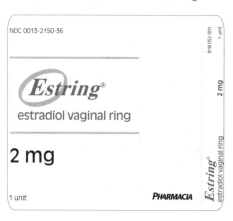

Source: © Pfizer Inc. Used with permission.

67. Circle the control number of the drug on the label provided.

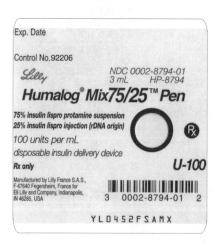

Source: © Eli Lilly and Company. Used with permission.

68. Circle the directions for diluting and mixing the drug on the label provided.

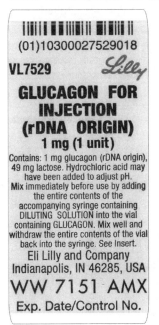

69. Circle the name of the manufacturing company that makes the drug on the label provided.

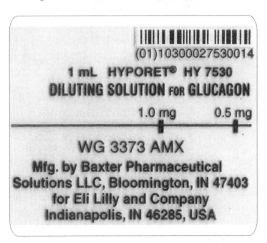

70. When using an insulin syringe, how many units of insulin would you have if you were to draw 1.5 ml of medication using the label provided? _____ units

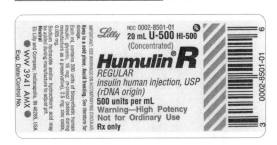

71. A patient is to receive 50 units of insulin every morning. How many days would the KwikPen last based on the information provided on the drug label? _____ days

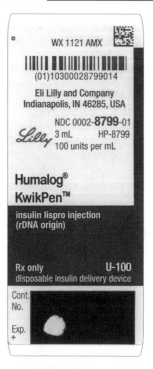

72. A client is to self-administer 22 units of insulin. Using the drug label provided, calculate how many ml the client should draw into a U-100 insulin syringe. _____ ml

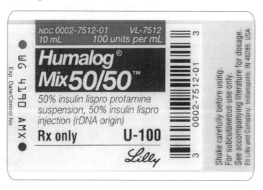

73. Circle the expiration date of the drug on the label provided.

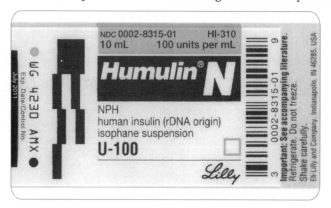

74. A healthcare provider draws the entire contents of the medication based on the label provided. If the healthcare provider has drawn 3 ml, how many units of insulin is he or she prepared to administer? _____ units

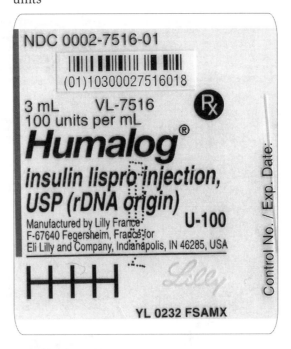

75. Circle the number of doses of the drug using the label provided.

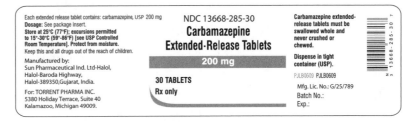

76. Circle the directions for taking the drug using the label provided.

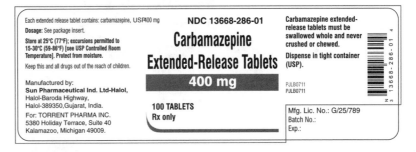

77. A client takes 20 mg of citalopram hydrobromide QID. Using the label provided, calculate how many days the client will take the medication before finishing the prescription. _____ days

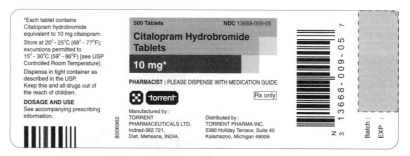

Source: © Torrent Pharma Inc. Used with permission.

78. A client is taking sertraline hydrochloride 100 mg po every day. Using the label provided, how many tablets should she be instructed to pour? _____ tablets

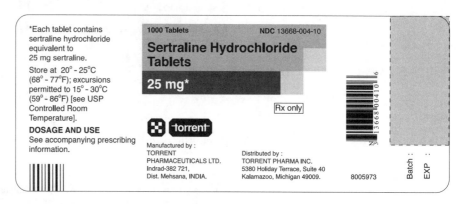

Source: © Torrent Pharma Inc. Used with permission.

79. Circle the bar code on the drug label provided.

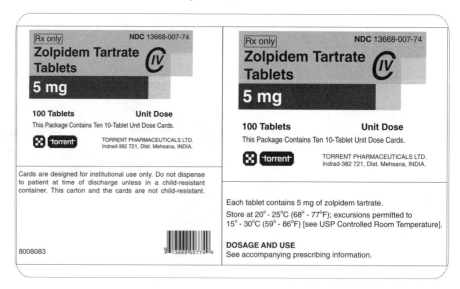

Source: © Torrent Pharma Inc. Used with permission.

80. Circle the drug use on the label provided.

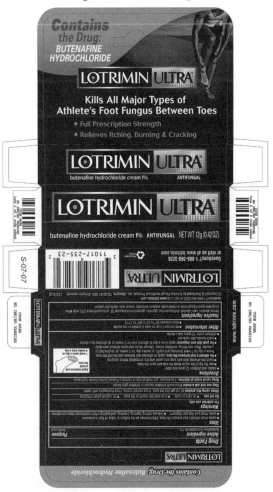

81. Circle the dosage supplied of the drug using the label provided.

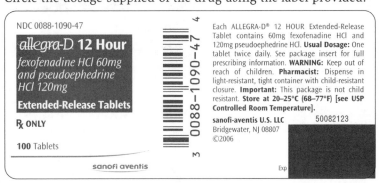

82. What is the generic name of the drug listed on the label provided?

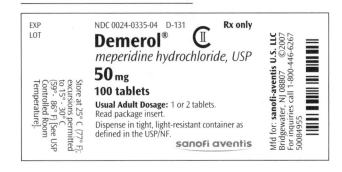

83. Using the label provided, determine how much furosemide each Lasix tablet contains. _____

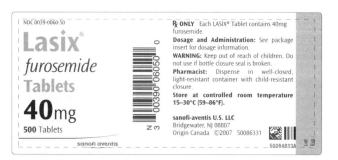

Source: © sanofi-aventis US. Used with permission.

84. Circle the dose strength of the drug using the label provided.

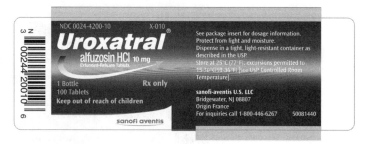

Source: © sanofi-aventis US. Used with permission.

85. A client has this IV hung at 7 am and it is set to run at 125 ml/hr. At 11 am the IV is checked to determine the amount of fluid left in the bag. Using the label provided, calculate the amount of fluid infused and shade the picture with the amount of fluid remaining.

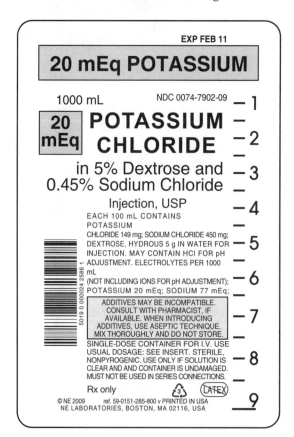

86. Identify the number of units shaded in the insulin syringe: _____ units

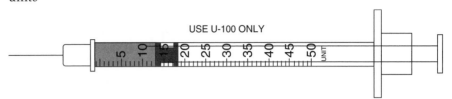

87. Identify the number of milliliters shaded in the standard syringe: _____ milliliters

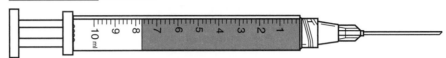

88. Identify the number of milliliters shaded in the standard syringe: _____ milliliters

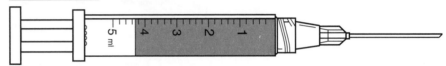

89. Identify the number of minims shaded in the tuberculin syringe: _____ minims

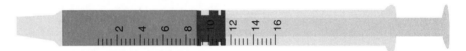

90. Identify the number of milliliters shaded in the standard syringe: _____ milliliters

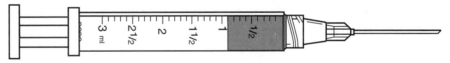

91. Identify the number of milliliters shaded in the standard syringe: _____ milliliters

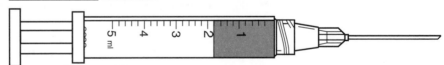

92. Identify the number of minims shaded in the tuberculin syringe: _____ minims

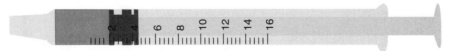

93. Identify the number of units shaded in the insulin syringe: _____ units

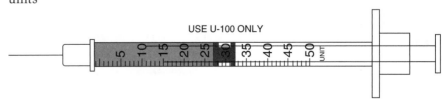

94. Identify the number of milliliters shaded in the standard syringe: _____ milliliters

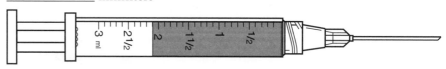

95. Identify the number of milliliters shaded in the standard syringe: _____ milliliters

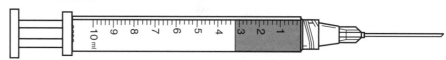

96. Identify the number of minims shaded in the tuberculin syringe: _____ minims

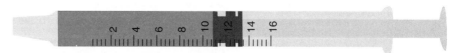

97. Identify the number of milliliters shaded in the standard syringe: _____ milliliters

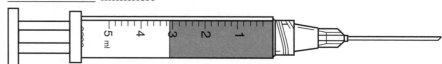

98. Identify the number of milliliters shaded in the standard syringe: _____ milliliters

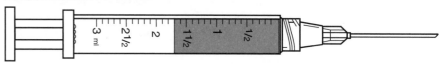

99. Identify the number of milliliters shaded in the standard syringe: _____ milliliters

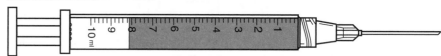

100. Identify the number of units shaded in the insulin syringe: _____ units

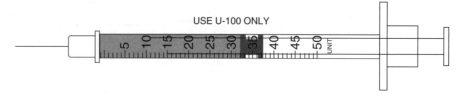

Answers to Comprehensive Examination I

1. 1 g
2. 21 gtts/min; 125 ml/hr
3. gr I
4. 2.5 ml

   Ratio and proportion method:

   1 g : 5 ml :: 500 mg : x ml = 2.5 ml

   $$\frac{1\,g}{5\,ml} = \frac{0.5\,g}{x\,ml} = 2.5\,ml$$

Dosage formula method:

$$\frac{500 \text{ mg}}{1000 \text{ mg}} \times 5 \text{ ml} = 2.5 \text{ ml}$$

Dimensional analysis method:

$$x \text{ ml} = \frac{5 \text{ ml}}{1000 \text{ mg}} \times \frac{500 \text{ mg}}{1} = 2.5 \text{ ml}$$

5. 13.6 kg

   204 mg; 20.4 ml

   5 ml po QID

6. 60 gtts

7. 1000 ml

8. 1 minim

9. 240 ml

10. 17 gtts/min

$$\frac{1000 \text{ ml}}{2 \text{ hr}} \times \frac{20 \text{ gtts/ml}}{60 \text{ min}} = 17 \text{ gtts/min}$$

50 ml/hr

$$\frac{1000 \text{ ml}}{2 \text{ hr}} = 50 \text{ ml/hr}$$

11. 5 ml

    75 gtts/min

$$\frac{50 \text{ mg}}{20 \text{ min}} \times \frac{15 \text{ gtts/ml}}{1} = 75 \text{ gtts/min}$$

If 100 ml must run in 20 min, then the rate must be 300 ml/hr (20 min $\times$ 3 = 60 min).

12. gr XV

13. 0.38

14. 0.8

15. 0.5

16. 0.9

17. 0.18

18. $^1/_3$

19. $^2/_3$

20. 4

21. CMCLXVIII

22. CIX

23. VIISS

24. DCL

25. CDXLIV

26. 3500 ml

27. 0.5 g

28. 1 pt

29. 66 oz

30. 1 fluidram
31. gr $^1/_{10}$
32. 8 drams
33. 2.2 lb
34. 1 lb
35. 60 minims
36. 1200 mg
37. 90 ml
38. 2 ml
39. 2 tablets (1 g = 1000 mg)
40. 3 tablets
41. 40 ml
42. a. Right drug
    b. Right dose
    c. Right route
    d. Right time
    e. Right client
    f. Right documentation
43. 50 gtts/min

$$\frac{250 \text{ ml}}{5 \text{ hr}} = 50 \text{ gtts/min}$$

50 ml/hr

$$\frac{250 \text{ ml}}{5 \text{ hr}} = 50 \text{ ml/hr}$$

44. 125 ml/hr

$$\frac{3000 \text{ ml}}{24 \text{ hr}} = 125 \text{ ml/hr}$$

45. 67 gtts/min

$$\frac{100 \text{ ml}}{30 \text{ min}} \times \frac{20 \text{ gtts/ml}}{1} = 67 \text{ gtts/min}$$

200 ml/hr

$$\frac{100 \text{ ml}}{0.5 \text{ hr}} = 200 \text{ ml/hr}$$

46. 108 ml/hr

$$\frac{325 \text{ ml}}{3 \text{ hr}} = 108 \text{ ml/hr}$$

47. 74 inches, 185 cm
48. 95.4 kg
49. 63 inches, 157.5 cm
50. 54.5 kg
51. $^1/_2$ tablet

Grain 1 = 60 mg

Ratio and proportion method:

60 mg : 1 tablet :: 30 mg : x tablets = $^1\!/_2$ tablet

$$\frac{60\ mg}{1\ tablet} = \frac{30\ mg}{x\ tablet} = 0.5\ tablet$$

Dosage formula method:

$$\frac{30\ mg}{60\ mg} \times 1\ tablet = 0.5\ tablet = \tfrac{1}{2}\ tablet$$

Dimensional analysis method:

$$x\ tablets = \frac{1\ tablet}{60\ mg} \times \frac{30\ mg}{1}\, 30\ mg/1 = 0.5\ tablet = \tfrac{1}{2}\ tablet$$

52. gr $^1\!/_4$

53. 63 gtts/min

$$\frac{500\ ml}{120\ min} \times \frac{15\ gtts/ml}{1} = 62.5\ gtts/min$$

250 ml/hr

$$\frac{500\ ml}{2\ hr} = 250\ ml/hr$$

54. 0.5 ml

200 gtts/min

$$\frac{50\ ml}{15\ min} \times \frac{60}{1} = 200\ gtts/min$$

200 ml/hr

50 ml : 15 min :: x ml : 60 min = 200 ml/hr

(With microtubing, the ml/hr are the same as the gtts/min.)

55. 17 gtts/min

$$\frac{200\ ml}{2\ hr} \times \frac{10\ gtts/ml}{60min} = 16.6\ gtts/min$$

100 ml/hr

$$\frac{200\ ml}{2\ hr} = 100\ ml/hr$$

56.

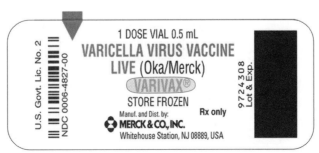

57.

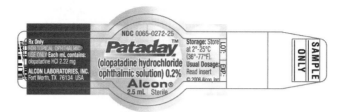

Source: © Alcon Laboratories, Inc. Used with permission.

58.

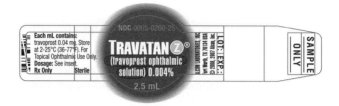

Source: © Alcon Laboratories, Inc. Used with permission.

59.

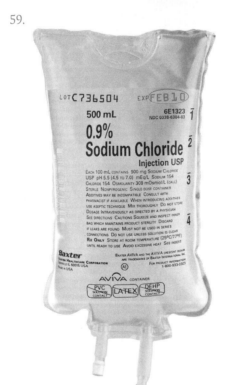

Source: © Baxter Healthcare Corporation. Used with permission.

60.

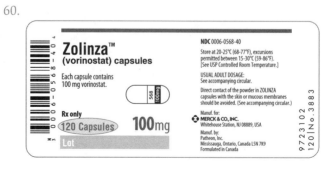

Source: Courtesy of Merck & Co., Inc.

61.

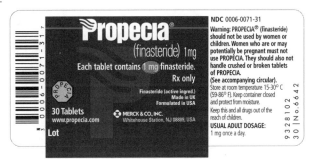

62.

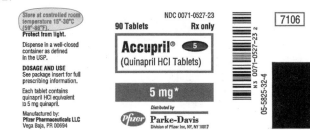

63. **2 tablets**

$$\frac{0.5 \text{ mg}}{0.25 \text{ mg}} \times 1 \text{ tablet} = 2 \text{ tablets}$$

64.

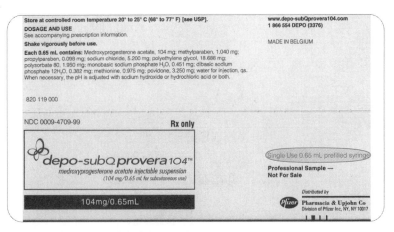

65.

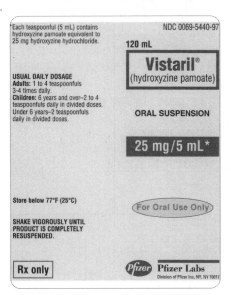

66.

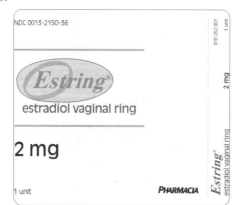

Source: © Pfizer Inc. Used with permission.

67.

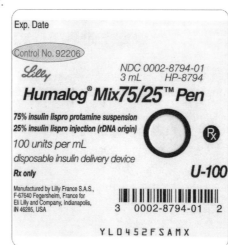

Source: © Eli Lilly and Company. Used with permission.

68.

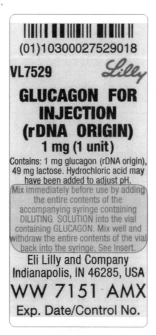

Source: © Eli Lilly and Company. Used with permission.

69.

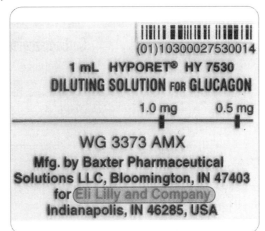

70. 750 units

71. 6 days

$$100 \text{ units per ml}, 3 \text{ ml} = 300 \text{ units}, 50 \text{ units per day}, \frac{300 \text{ units}}{50 \text{ units}} = 6 \text{ days}$$

72. 0.22 ml

$$\frac{22 \text{ units}}{100 \text{ units}} \times 1 \text{ ml} = 0.22 \text{ ml}$$

73.

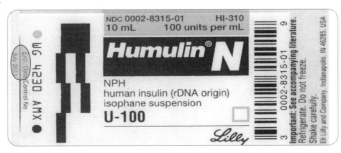

74. 300 units

100 units : 1 ml :: x units : 3 ml = 300 units

75.

76.

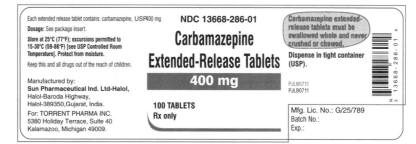

77. 62.5 days

$$\frac{500 \text{ tablets}}{8 \text{ tablets/day}} = 62.5 \text{ days}$$

78. 4 tablets

$$\frac{100 \text{ mg}}{25 \text{ mg}} \times 1 \text{ tablet} = 4 \text{ tablets}$$

79.

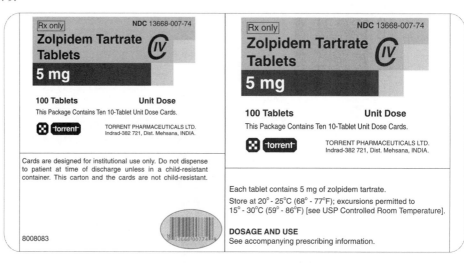

80.

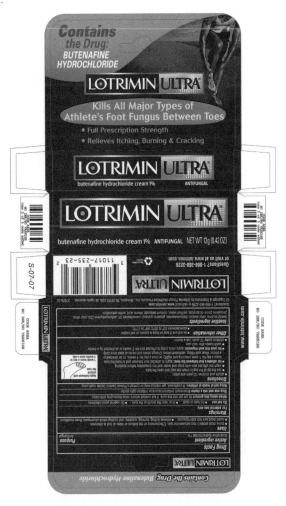

Source: The Lotrimin Ultra® and
Claritin® labels are reproduced with
permission of Schering Corporation.
All rights reserved. Lotrimin
Ultra and Claritin are registered
trademarks of Schering Corporation.

81.

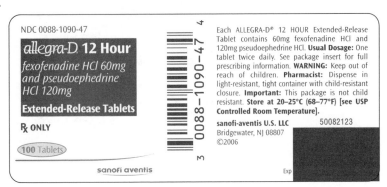

Source: © sanofi-aventis US. Used with
permission.

82. Meperidine hydrochloride
83. 40 mg
84.

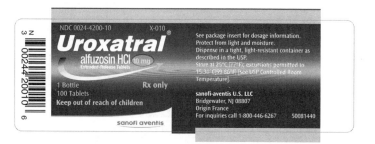

Source: © sanofi-aventis US. Used with permission.

85.

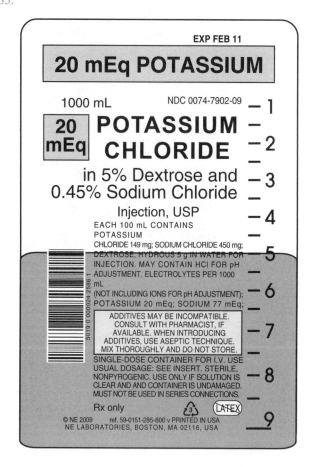

500 ml infused: 125 ml × 4 hours = 500 ml

500 ml left in bag (LIB): 1000 ml − 500 ml = 500 ml

86. 13 units
87. 7.7 ml
88. 4.3 ml
89. 9 minims
90. 0.9 ml
91. 1.8 ml
92. 2 minims

93. 27 units
94. 2.1 ml
95. 3.2 ml
96. 11 minims
97. 3.1 ml
98. 1.7 ml
99. 8.1 ml
100. 32 units

10 Comprehensive Examination II

Unless otherwise instructed, answer the questions by filling in the missing information. Be sure to show all your work and to proof all answers.

1. 750 mg = _____ g

2. The MD orders an IV of 500 ml D&0.225NS to infuse in 8 hr. The drop factor on the tubing is 15 gtts/ml. Give:

   _____ gtts/min   _____ ml/hr

3. 15 mg = gr _____

4. The MD orders 25 mg of a medication. On hand is 0.1 g of the medication in 10 ml. Give: _____

   Solve using the following three methods.

   Ratio and proportion method:

   Dosage formula method:

   Dimensional analysis method:

5. A toddler weighs 25 lb and has an order for amoxicillin 35 mg po QID. The safe dosage range for this medication is 5 mg/kg/QID. The supply is 5 mg/1 ml oral suspension. *Calculate:*

   25 lb = _____ kg

   The safe dosage limit per day: _____ mg or _____ ml

   Give: _____ ml po QID

6. 1 tbs = _____ ml

7. 500 ml = _____ pt

8. gr $^1/_{300}$ = _____ mg

9. 30 g = _____ drams

10. The MD orders 1000 ml D5W with 100 units regular insulin to run at 5 units per hr. The drop factor on the tubing is 60 gtts/ml. *Calculate:*

    _____ gtts/min   _____ ml/hr

11. The anesthesiologist has ordered morphine 10 mg IVPB Q4H PRN for pain for a postoperative cholecystectomy client. The supply is 5 mg/1 ml in a 5-ml vial. The nurse prepares the IBPB with 100 ml NS to infuse in 30 min. The drop factor on the tubing is 10 gtts/ml. *Calculate*:

    Morphine 10 mg = _____ ml

    _____ gtts/min   _____ ml/hr

12. gr XXV = _____ mg

For questions 13–17, convert to decimals.

13. $^6/_7$ = _____
14. $^1/_4$ = _____
15. $^2/_9$ = _____
16. $^6/_{36}$ = _____
17. $^3/_4$ = _____

For questions 18–20, solve and reduce the following to the lowest form.

18. $^5/_{35}$ = _____
19. $^2/_5 + ^4/_5$ = _____
20. $^3/_4 - ^1/_2$ = _____

For questions 21–25, convert to Roman numerals.

21. 1842 = _____
22. 111 = _____
23. 35.5 = _____
24. 700 = _____
25. 27 = _____
26. 6.4 L = _____ ml
27. 750 mg = _____ g
28. 480 ml = _____ pt
29. gr $^1/_4$ = _____ mg
30. 3 tbs = _____ ml
31. 6.6 lb = _____ kg
32. 8 oz = _____ ml
33. gr $^1/_{150}$ = _____ g
34. gr $^1/_{100}$ = _____ mg
35. 900 g = _____ lb
36. Height: 6 ft 4 in = _____ in = _____ cm
37. Weight: 190 lb = _____ kg
38. Height: 5 ft 0 in = _____ in = _____ cm
39. Weight: 103 lb = _____ kg
40. An IV of 1000 ml D5W hung at 10 am has 400 ml LIB. The doctor orders the remaining fluid to be infused in 3 hr. The drop factor on the tubing is 20 gtts/ml. At what rate should the nurse set the infusion pump?

    _____ ml/hr

41. 15 mg : gr $^1/_4$ :: x mg : gr $^3/_4$ = _____ mg
42. 5 ml : 1 tsp :: x ml : 4 tsp = _____ ml
43. 20 ml : 1 g :: x ml : 1500 mg = _____ ml

44. $\dfrac{100\ mg}{250\ mg} \times 2\ ml = $ _____ ml

45. x capsules $= \dfrac{1\ capsule}{100\ mg} \times \dfrac{200\ mg}{1} = $ _____ capsules

46. x ml $= \dfrac{20\ ml}{40\ mEq} \times \dfrac{15\ mEq}{1} = $ _____ ml

47. List four of the six guidelines in preventing medication administration errors.

    a.

    b.

    c.

    d.

    e. (optional)

    f. (optional)

48. The MD orders 500 ml RL IV to infuse in 5 hr. The drop factor on the tubing is 60 gtts/ml. *Calculate:*

    _____ gtts/min   _____ ml/hr

49. The MD orders 1000 ml D5W with 40 meq KCL to run at 5 mEq/hr. The drop factor on the tubing is 15 gtts/ml. *Calculate:*

    _____ gtts/min   _____ ml/hr

50. The MD orders Lasix (furosemide) 20 mg IVPB STAT. The nurse prepares a 50-ml IVPB of NS to run in 15 min. Microtubing is used. *Calculate:*

    _____ gtts/min   _____ ml/hr

51. The MD orders 0.125 mg of a medication. The supply is 0.25-mg scored tablets.

    Give: _____

    Solve using the following three methods.

    Ratio and proportion method:

    Dosage formula method:

    Dimensional analysis method:

52. 45 mg = gr _____

53. The doctor orders 250 ml NS IV with 10,000 units of heparin to run in 3 hr. The drop factor on the tubing is 20 gtts/ml. *Calculate:*

    _____ gtts/min   _____ ml/hr

54. The nurse anesthetist orders Stadol 2 mg IVPB Q4H PRN for pain for a postoperative client. The supply is 1 mg/0.5 ml in a 2-ml vial. The postanesthesia care nurse prepares the IVPB with 100 ml NS to run in 20 min. Drop factor on the tubing is 10 gtts/ml. *Calculate:*

    Stadol 2 mg = _____ ml

    _____ gtts/min   _____ ml/hr

55. A client scheduled for transfer to a skilled nursing facility has 100 ml of D5W left in her IV bag at 9:30 am. The social worker tells you the ambulette is picking up the client at 12 noon. The MD writes an order to infuse the remaining fluid and discontinue the line. The drop factor on the tubing is 20 gtts/ml. At what rate should the nurse infuse the fluid? *Calculate*:

_____ gtts/min   _____ ml/hr

56. Circle the generic name of the drug using the label provided.

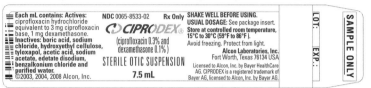

Source: © Alcon Laboratories, Inc. Used with permission.

57. Circle the brand name of the drug using the label provided.

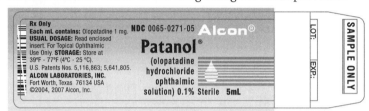

Source: © Alcon Laboratories, Inc. Used with permission.

58. Circle the supply dosage of the drug using the label provided.

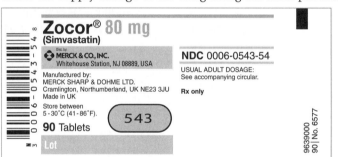

Source: Courtesy of Merck & Co., Inc.

59. Circle the amount of IV fluid in the bag using the label provided.

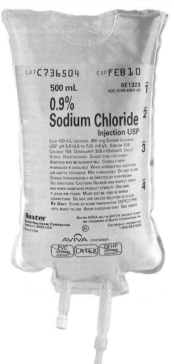

Source: © Baxter Healthcare Corporation. Used with permission.

60. Circle the lot number of the drug using the label provided.

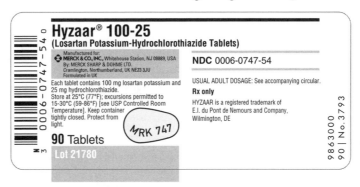

61. Circle the route of administration for the drug using the label provided.

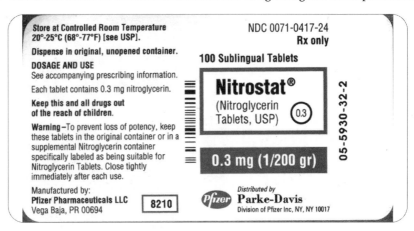

62. Circle the dosing instructions for client complaints using the drug label provided.

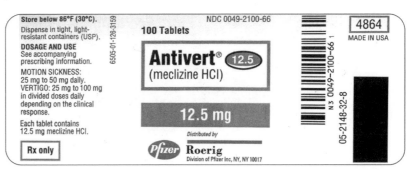

63. A client is to take 100 mg of Vibramycin po every day. Using the label provided, calculate what the client should take every day.

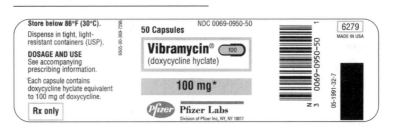

64. Circle the dosage supply of the drug using the label provided.

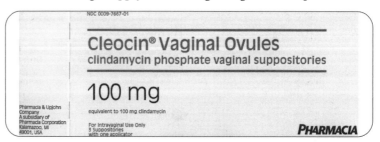

65. Circle the name of the drug manufacturer using the label provided.

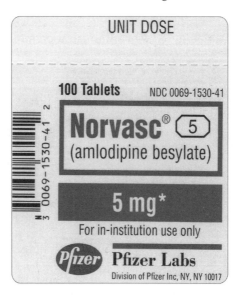

66. Circle the bar code of the drug using the label provided.

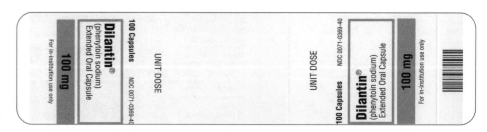

67. Circle the expiration date of the drug using the label provided.

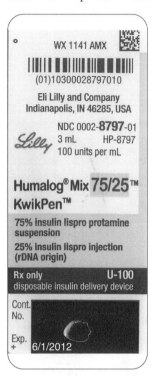

Source: © Eli Lilly and Company. Used with permission.

68. Circle the route instructions for the drug using the label provided.

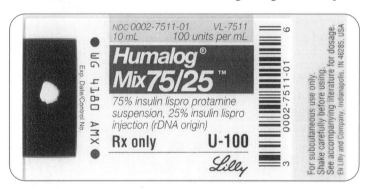

Source: © Eli Lilly and Company. Used with permission.

69. Circle the storage instructions for the drug using the label provided.

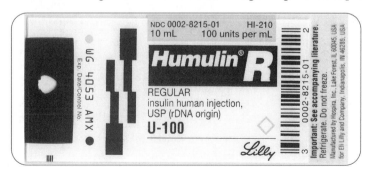

Source: © Eli Lilly and Company. Used with permission.

70. A client needs to take 50 units of insulin lispro every morning. Using the drug label provided, calculate what the client should take every morning.

_____

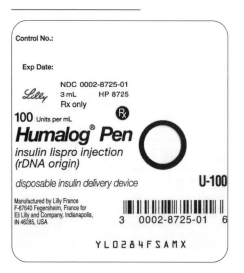

Source: © Eli Lilly and Company. Used with permission.

71. What is the percentage of human insulin injection contained in the vial according to the label provided? _____

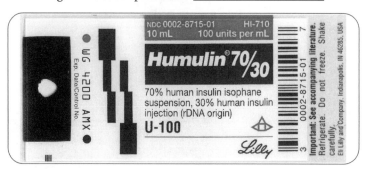

Source: © Eli Lilly and Company. Used with permission.

72. Circle the supply dose of the drug using the label provided.

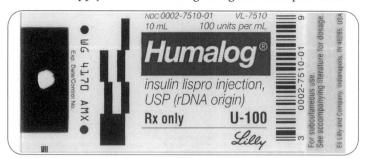

Source: © Eli Lilly and Company. Used with permission.

73. What is the total amount of insulin units in the container using the drug label provided? _____

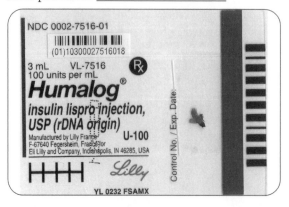

Source: © Eli Lilly and Company. Used with permission.

74. Circle the bar code for the drug using the label provided.

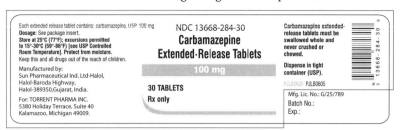

75. Using the label provided, how many milligrams of carbamazepine would a client take in total if the client took 4 tablets of the drug?

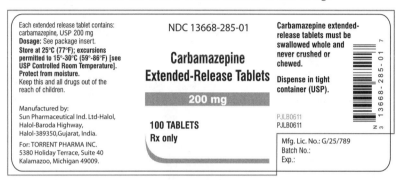

76. Circle the expiration date of the drug using the label provided.

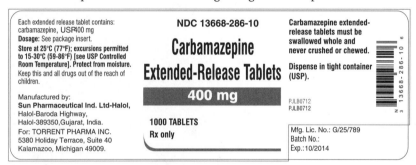

77. Circle the directions for the pharmacist according to the label provided.

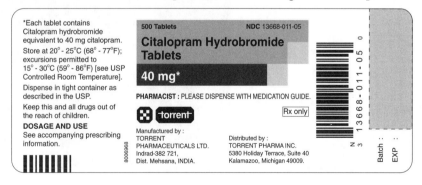

78. Circle the name of the distributor of the drug using the label provided.

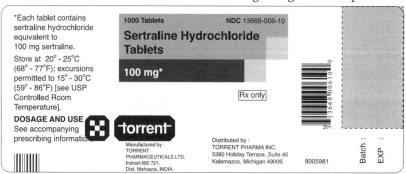

79. Circle the use of the drug using the label provided.

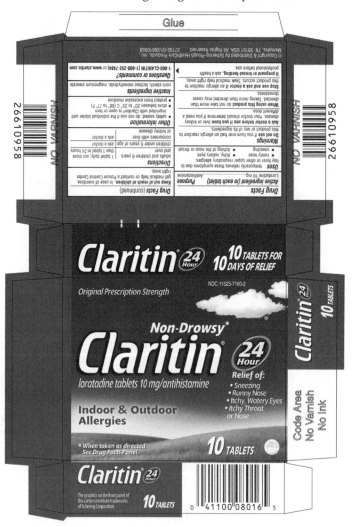

80. Circle the trade name of the drug using the label provided.

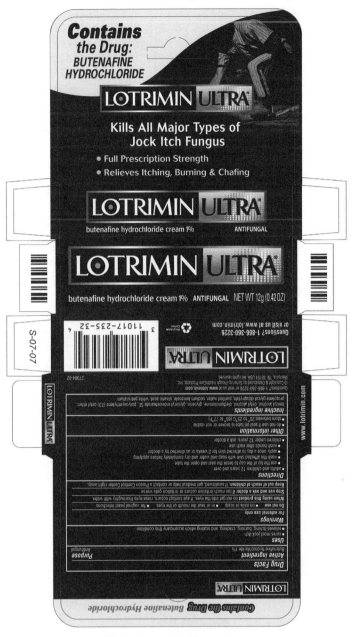

81. Circle the dosage of the drug using the label provided.

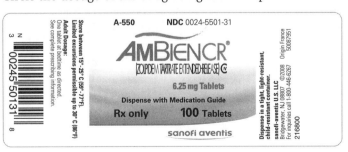

82. Circle the route of the drug using the label provided.

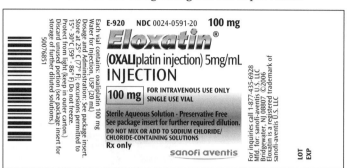

Source: © sanofi-aventis US. Used with permission.

83. Circle the generic name of the drug using the label provided.

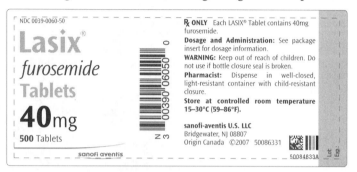

Source: © sanofi-aventis US. Used with permission.

84. Circle the dosage supply of the drug using the label provided.

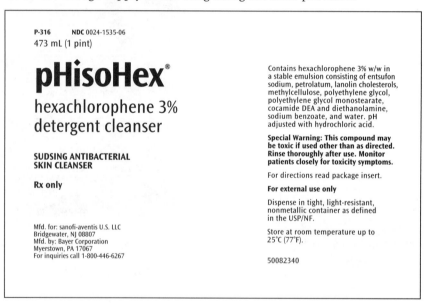

Source: © sanofi-aventis US. Used with permission.

85. Using the IV label provided, calculate the ml/hr and gtts/min for a client receiving 1 mEq of potassium every hour. Drop factor: 15.

_____ ml/hr _____ gtts/min

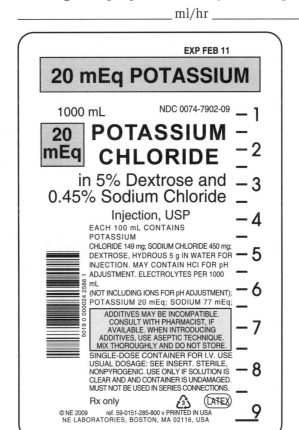

EXP FEB 11

20 mEq POTASSIUM

1000 mL   NDC 0074-7902-09   – 1

**20
mEq** **POTASSIUM** –
CHLORIDE – 2

in 5% Dextrose and – 3
0.45% Sodium Chloride –

Injection, USP – 4

EACH 100 mL CONTAINS
POTASSIUM
CHLORIDE 149 mg; SODIUM CHLORIDE 450 mg; –
DEXTROSE, HYDROUS 5 g IN WATER FOR – 5
INJECTION. MAY CONTAIN HCl FOR pH
ADJUSTMENT. ELECTROLYTES PER 1000
mL – 6
(NOT INCLUDING IONS FOR pH ADJUSTMENT);
POTASSIUM 20 mEq; SODIUM 77 mEq;

ADDITIVES MAY BE INCOMPATIBLE.
CONSULT WITH PHARMACIST, IF
AVAILABLE. WHEN INTRODUCING – 7
ADDITIVES, USE ASEPTIC TECHNIQUE.
MIX THOROUGHLY AND DO NOT STORE.

SINGLE-DOSE CONTAINER FOR I.V. USE
USUAL DOSAGE: SEE INSERT. STERILE, – 8
NONPYROGENIC. USE ONLY IF SOLUTION IS
CLEAR AND AND CONTAINER IS UNDAMAGED.
MUST NOT BE USED IN SERIES CONNECTIONS.

Rx only   (LATEX)
© NE 2009   ref. 59-0151-285-800 v PRINTED IN USA – 9
NE LABORATORIES, BOSTON, MA 02116, USA

86. Identify the number of units shaded in the insulin syringe: _____ units

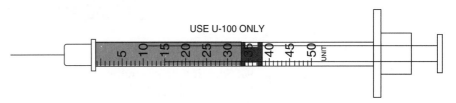

USE U-100 ONLY

87. Identify the number of milliliters shaded in the standard syringe: _____ milliliters

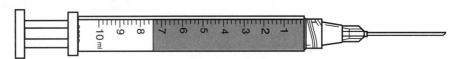

88. Identify the number of milliliters shaded in the standard syringe: _____ milliliters

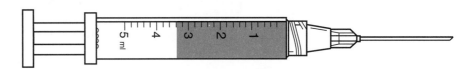

89. Identify the number of minims shaded in the tuberculin syringe: _____ minims

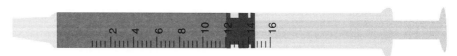

90. Identify the number of milliliters shaded in the standard syringe: _____ milliliters

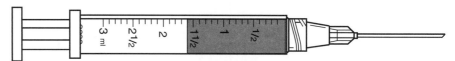

91. Identify the number of milliliters shaded in the standard syringe: _____ milliliters

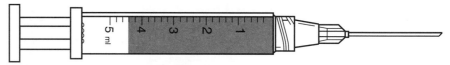

92. Identify the number of minims shaded in the tuberculin syringe: _____ minims

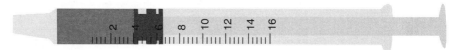

93. Identify the number of units shaded in the insulin syringe: _____ units

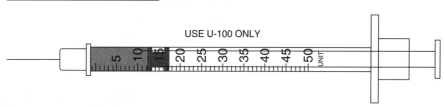

94. Identify the number of milliliters shaded in the standard syringe: _____ milliliters

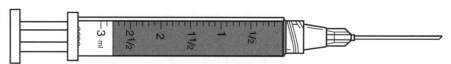

95. Identify the number of milliliters shaded in the standard syringe: _____ milliliters

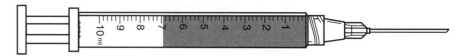

96. Identify the number of minims shaded in the tuberculin syringe: _____ minims

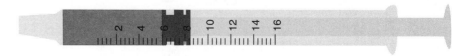

97. Identify the number of milliliters shaded in the standard syringe: _____ milliliters

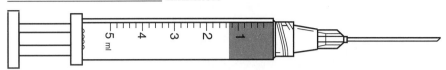

98. Identify the number of milliliters shaded in the standard syringe: _____ milliliters

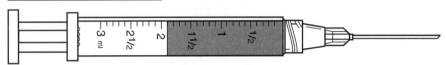

99. Identify the number of milliliters shaded in the standard syringe: _____ milliliters

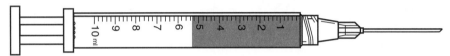

100. Identify the number of units shaded in the insulin syringe: _____ units

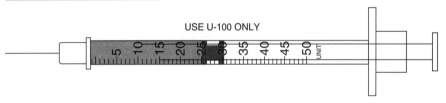

Answers to Comprehensive Examination II

1. 0.75 g
2. 16 gtts/min

$$\frac{500 \text{ ml}}{8 \text{ hr}} \times \frac{15 \text{ gtts/ml}}{60 \text{ min}} = 15.6 \text{ gtts/min} = 16 \text{ gtts/min}$$

63 ml/hr

$$\frac{500 \text{ ml}}{8 \text{ hr}} = 62.5 \text{ ml/hr}$$

3. gr $^1/_4$
4. 2.5 ml

Ratio and proportion method:

0.1 g : 10 ml :: 25 mg : x ml = 2.5 ml

$$\frac{100 \text{ mg}}{10 \text{ ml}} = \frac{25 \text{ mg}}{x \text{ ml}} = 2.5 \text{ ml}$$

Dosage formula method:

$$\frac{25 \text{ mg}}{100 \text{ mg}} \times 10 \text{ ml} = 2.5 \text{ ml}$$

Dimensional analysis method:

$$x \text{ ml} = \frac{10 \text{ ml}}{100 \text{ mg}} \times \frac{25 \text{ mg}}{1} = 2.5 \text{ ml}$$

5. 11.3 kg

   56.5 mg; 11.3 ml

   7 ml po QID

6. 15 ml

7. 1 pt

8. 0.2 mg

9. 8 drams

10. 50 gtts/min; 50 ml/hr

11. 2 ml

   $$\frac{10\,mg}{5\,mg} \times 1\,ml = 2\,ml$$

   33 gtts/min

   $$\frac{10\,mg}{30\,min} \times \frac{10}{1} = \frac{1000}{30} = 33.3 = 33\,gtts/min$$

   200 ml/hr

   100 ml : 30 min :: x ml : 60 min = 200 ml/hr

12. 1500 mg

13. 0.85

14. 0.25

15. 0.22

16. 0.16

17. 0.75

18. $^1/_7$

19. $1^1/_5$

20. $^1/_4$

21. MDCCCXLII

22. CXI

23. XXXV$\overline{ss}$

24. DCC

25. XXVII

26. 6400 ml

27. 0.75 g

28. 1 pt

29. 15 mg

30. 45 ml

31. 3 kg

32. 240 ml

33. 0.0004 g

34. 0.6 mg

35. 1.98 lb = 2 lb

36. 76 in, 190 cm

37. 86.3 kg

38. 60 in, 150 cm

39. 46.8 kg

40. 133 ml/hr

41. 45 mg

42. 20 ml

43. 30 ml (Convert 1 g to 1000 mg)

44. 0.8 ml

45. 2 capsules

46. 7.5 ml

47. a. Read all labels carefully.

    b. Double-check large quantities of pills and liquids.

    c. Never guess with illegible handwriting.

    d. Look up new or unfamiliar medications.

    e. Properly identify all clients.

    f. Double-check all calculations.

48. 100 gtts/min

$$\frac{500 \text{ ml}}{5 \text{ hr}} = 100 \text{ gtts/min}$$

    100 ml/hr

$$\frac{500 \text{ ml}}{5 \text{ hr}} = 100 \text{ ml/hr}$$

49. 31 gtts/min

$$\frac{125 \text{ ml}}{60} \times \frac{15}{1} = 31 \text{ gtts/min}$$

    125 ml/hr

    40 mEq : 1000 ml :: 5 mEq : x ml $= 125$ ml/hour

50. 200 gtts/min

$$\frac{50 \text{ ml}}{0.25 \text{ hr}} \times \frac{60}{60} = 200 \text{ gtts/min}$$

    200 ml/hr

$$\frac{50 \text{ ml}}{0.25 \text{ hr}} = 200 \text{ ml/hr}$$

51. $^{1}/_{2}$ tablet

    Ratio and proportion method:

    0.25 mg : 1 tablet :: 0.125 mg : x tablets $= ^{1}/_{2}$ tablet

$$\frac{0.25 \text{ mg}}{1 \text{ tablet}} = \frac{0.125 \text{ mg}}{x \text{ tablet}} = \tfrac{1}{2} \text{ tablet}$$

    Dosage formula method:

$$\frac{0.125 \text{ mg}}{0.25 \text{ mg}} \times 1 \text{ tablet} = \tfrac{1}{2} \text{ tablet}$$

    Dimensional anlysis method:

$$x \text{ tablets} = \frac{1 \text{ tablet}}{0.25 \text{ mg}} \times \frac{0.125 \text{ mg}}{1} = \tfrac{1}{2} \text{ tablet}$$

52. gr $^3/_4$

53. 28 gtts/min

$$\frac{250 \text{ ml}}{3 \text{ hr}} \times \frac{20 \text{ gtts/ml}}{60 \text{ min}} = 27.7 \text{ gtts/min}$$

83 ml/hr

$$\frac{250 \text{ ml}}{3 \text{ hr}} = 83.3 \text{ ml/hr}$$

54. 1 ml Stadol (1 mg/0.5 ml × 2)

50 gtts/min

$$\frac{100 \text{ ml}}{20 \text{ min}} \times \frac{10 \text{ gtts/ml}}{1} = 50 \text{ gtts/min}$$

300 ml/hr (100 ml/hr for 20 min × 3)

55. 13 gtts/min

$$\frac{100 \text{ ml}}{2.5 \text{ hr}} \times \frac{20 \text{ gtts/ml}}{60 \text{ min}} = 13.3 \text{ gtts/min}$$

40 ml/hr

$$\frac{100 \text{ ml}}{2.5 \text{ hr}} = 40 \text{ ml/hr}$$

56.

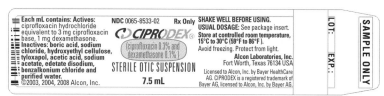

Source: © Alcon Laboratories, Inc. Used with permission.

57.

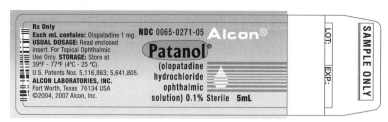

Source: © Alcon Laboratories, Inc. Used with permission.

58.

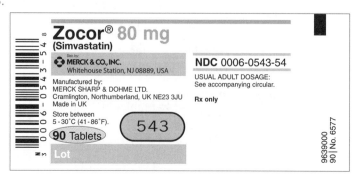

Source: Courtesy of Merck & Co., Inc.

59.

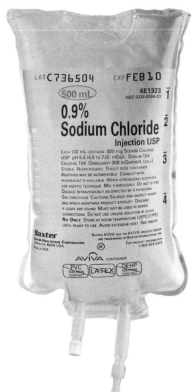

Source: © Baxter Healthcare
Corporation. Used with permission.

60.

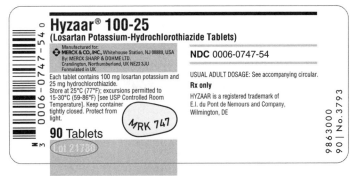

Source: Courtesy of Merck & Co.,
Inc.

61.

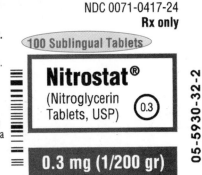

Source: © Pfizer Inc. Used with
permission.

62.

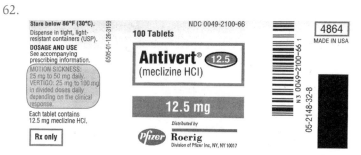

63. 1 capsule

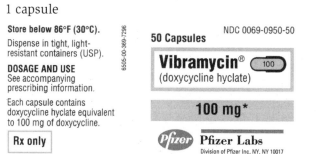

64.

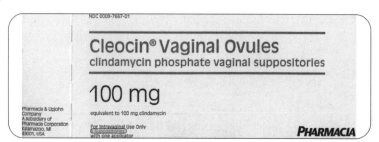

65.

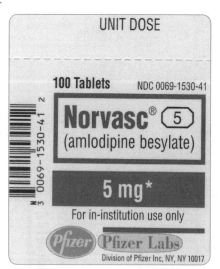

66.

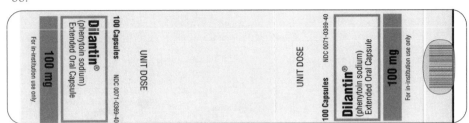

67.

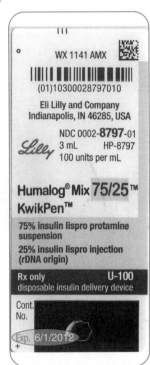

68.

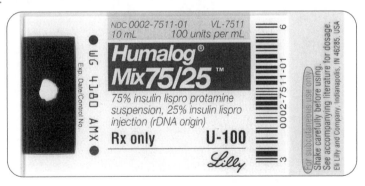

69.

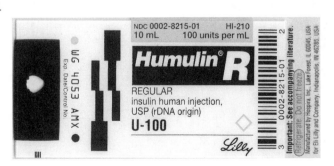

70. 0.5 ml

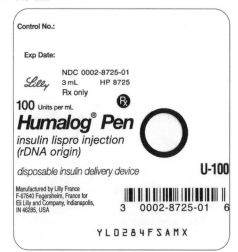

71. 30% human insulin injection

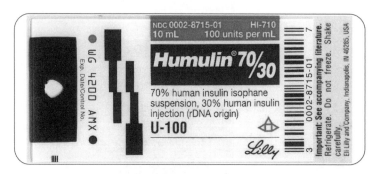

72.

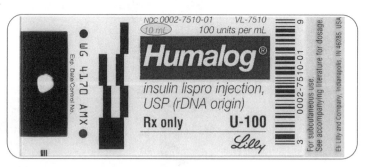

73. 300 units

74.

Each extended release tablet contains: carbamazepine, USP100 mg
Dosage: See package insert.
Store at 25°C (77°F); excursions permitted to 15°-30°C (59°-86°F) [see USP Controlled Room Temperature]. Protect from moisture.
Keep this and all drugs out of the reach of children.

Manufactured by:
Sun Pharmaceutical Ind. Ltd-Halol,
Halol-Baroda Highway,
Halol-389350,Gujarat, India.

For: TORRENT PHARMA INC.
5380 Holiday Terrace, Suite 40
Kalamazoo, Michigan 49009.

NDC 13668-284-30
Carbamazepine
Extended-Release Tablets
100 mg

30 TABLETS
Rx only

Carbamazepine extended-release tablets must be swallowed whole and never crushed or chewed.

Dispense in tight container (USP).

PJLB0605 PJLB0605

Mfg. Lic. No.: G/25/789
Batch No.:
Exp.:

75. **800 mg total**

76.

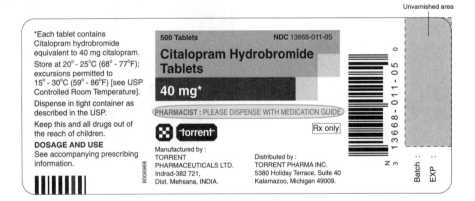

Each extended release tablet contains:
carbamazepine, USP400 mg
Dosage: See package insert.
Store at 25°C (77°F); excursions permitted to 15-30°C (59-86°F) [see USP Controlled Room Temperature]. Protect from moisture.
Keep this and all drugs out of the reach of children.

Manufactured by:
Sun Pharmaceutical Ind. Ltd-Halol,
Halol-Baroda Highway,
Halol-389350,Gujarat, India.
For: TORRENT PHARMA INC.
5380 Holiday Terrace, Suite 40
Kalamazoo, Michigan 49009.

NDC 13668-286-10
Carbamazepine
Extended-Release Tablets
400 mg

1000 TABLETS
Rx only

Carbamazepine extended-release tablets must be swallowed whole and never crushed or chewed.

Dispense in tight container (USP).

PJLB0712
PJLB0712

Mfg. Lic. No.: G/25/789
Batch No.:
Exp.: 10/2014

77.

Unvarnished area

*Each tablet contains Citalopram hydrobromide equivalent to 40 mg citalopram.
Store at 20° - 25°C (68° - 77°F); excursions permitted to 15° - 30°C (59° - 86°F) [see USP Controlled Room Temperature].
Dispense in tight container as described in the USP.
Keep this and all drugs out of the reach of children.
DOSAGE AND USE
See accompanying prescribing information.

500 Tablets   NDC 13668-011-05
Citalopram Hydrobromide Tablets
40 mg*

PHARMACIST : PLEASE DISPENSE WITH MEDICATION GUIDE.

torrent   Rx only

Manufactured by :
TORRENT
PHARMACEUTICALS LTD.
Indrad-382 721,
Dist. Mehsana, INDIA.

Distributed by :
TORRENT PHARMA INC.
5380 Holiday Terrace, Suite 40
Kalamazoo, Michigan 49009.

8006968

Batch :   EXP :

78.

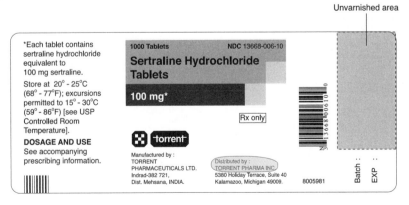

Unvarnished area

*Each tablet contains sertraline hydrochloride equivalent to 100 mg sertraline.
Store at 20° - 25°C (68° - 77°F); excursions permitted to 15° - 30°C (59° - 86°F) [see USP Controlled Room Temperature].
DOSAGE AND USE
See accompanying prescribing information.

1000 Tablets   NDC 13668-006-10
Sertraline Hydrochloride Tablets
100 mg*

Rx only

torrent

Manufactured by :
TORRENT
PHARMACEUTICALS LTD.
Indrad-382 721,
Dist. Mehsana, INDIA.

Distributed by :
TORRENT PHARMA INC.
5380 Holiday Terrace, Suite 40
Kalamazoo, Michigan 49009.

8005981

Batch :   EXP :

79.

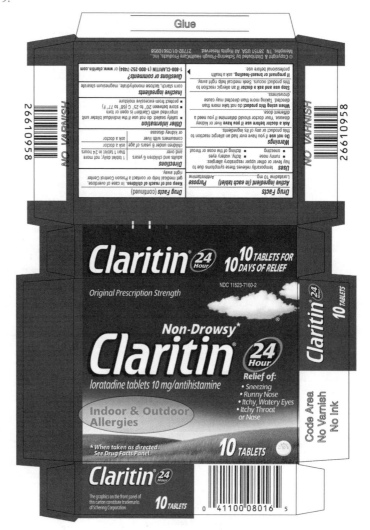

80.

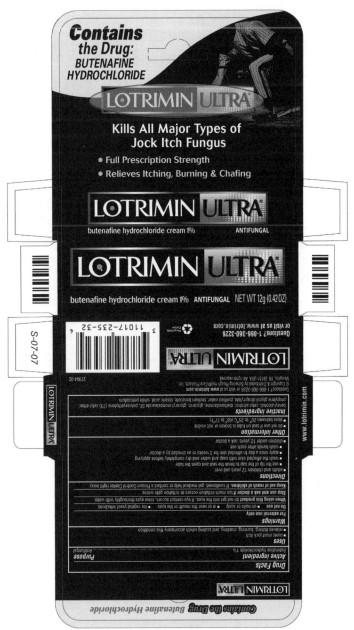

81.

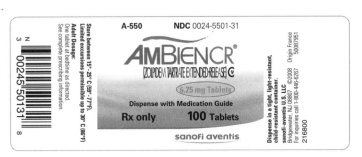

82.

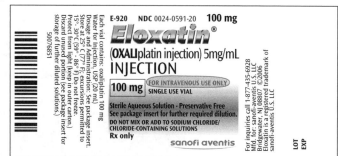

83.

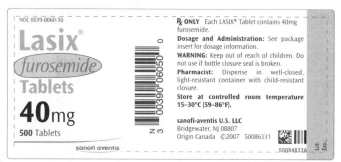

84.

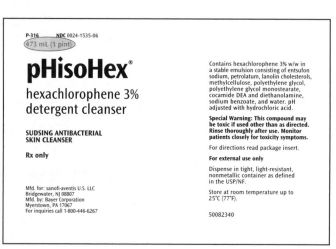

85. 100 ml/hr; 25 gtts/min

86. 33 units

87. 7.4 ml

88. 3.4 ml

89. 12 minims

90. 1.6 ml

91. 4.4 ml

92. 4 minims

93. 12 units

94. 2.8 ml

95. 6.9 ml

96. 6 minims

97. 1.3 ml

98. 1.9 ml

99. 5.3 ml

100. 25 units

Index

Locators in *italics* refer to selected Medication Administration Tips in the text.

Angeles College
3440 Wilshire Blvd., Suite 310
Los Angeles, CA 90010
Tel. (213) 487-2211